Women &
the Welfare State

TAVISTOCK WOMEN'S STUDIES

Women &
the Welfare State

ELIZABETH WILSON

TAVISTOCK PUBLICATIONS

London and New York

For Angela Weir. *This book is as much hers as mine. We discussed the subject in all its aspects while I was writing it, and before that, and in many places I am simply giving expression to her ideas.*

I am especially grateful to the following for their help and comments at various stages in the writing of this book: to the Red Rag Collective who first gave me the opportunity to develop my ideas in pamphlet form, and discussed them with me; to Gareth Stedman Jones, Ronnie Frankenberg, and Ian Gough; and to Mary McIntosh and the many other feminists with whom I have discussed these ideas. Since I have no wife, I am indebted only to myself for typing and general domestic servicing, although I am aware that those who were living with me while I was revising and typing the manuscript had to endure much moodiness and I am grateful for their forbearance. My thanks also to Jenny Morris for collating the Index.

First published in 1977 by
Tavistock Publications Limited
11 New Fetter Lane,
London EC4P 4EE
Reprinted 1982
Printed in Great Britain by
J. W. Arrowsmith Ltd
Bristol
Published in the USA by
Tavistock Publications in
association with Methuen, Inc.
733 Third Avenue,
New York, NY 10017

© *Elizabeth Wilson 1977*

ISBN 0 422 76050 1 *(hardbound)*
ISBN 0 422 76060 9 *(paperback)*

Contents

1 Introduction 7

2 Ideology & welfare 27

3 Women, social welfare, & social
  work in Victorian society 43

4 Women & the family since the
  Second World War 59

5 Welfare since the War 73

6 Welfare in the twentieth century 98

7 Welfare & war 126

8 Women & welfare: past & future 159

  References 188

  Subject Index 203

  Author Index 207

'A part of the bourgeoisie is desirous of redressing social griev-
ances, in order to secure the continued existence of bourgeois
society.
To this section belong economists, philanthropists, humani-
tarians, improvers of the condition of the working class, organ-
isers of charity, members of societies for the prevention of
cruelty to animals, temperance fanatics, hole-and-corner reformers of every imaginable kind. This form of Socialism has,
moreover, been worked out into complete systems . . .
The Socialistic bourgeois want all the advantages of modern
social conditions without the struggles and dangers necessarily
resulting therefrom. They desire the existing state of society
minus its revolutionary and disintegrating elements. They wish
for a bourgeoisie without a proletariat.'

Karl Marx and Frederick Engels : *Communist Manifesto*

ONE

Introduction

Feminism and socialism meet in the arena of the Welfare State, and the manipulations of the Welfare State offer a unique demonstration of how the State can prescribe what woman's consciousness should be. This book attempts to show that only a feminist analysis of the Welfare State that also relates it to a socialist perspective can enable us fully to understand why the conglomeration of legislation and services loosely labelled the Welfare State has come to be as it is. Only feminism has made it possible for us to see how the State defines femininity and that this definition is not marginal but is central to the purposes of welfarism. Woman is above all Mother, and with this vocation go all the virtues of femininity; submission, nurturance, passivity. The 'feminine' client of the social services waits patiently at clinics, social security offices, and housing departments, to be ministered to sometimes by the paternal authority figure, doctor or civil servant, sometimes by the nurturant yet firm model of femininity provided by nurse or social worker; in either case she goes away to do as she has been told – to take the pills, to love the baby.

The ways in which social policies discriminate against, or prescribe certain tasks and behaviours for women differ from the ways in which, say, pay structures or the law might be said to deny women a place in society equal to that of men. For it is quite widely recognized that the wage system discriminates against women and that the legal system continues to define women as the dependants of men in many areas of life. This recognition has recently been embodied in the *Equal Pay Act* (1970) and the *Sex Discrimination Act* (1975). As legislation they may be inadequate, but their existence proves that the problems are acknowledged. Welfare provision on the other hand operates in a more subtle and in some ways a more coercive fashion to keep women to their primary task as adults. This is the task of reproducing the work force. That the work force should be reproduced is obviously essential to the continuation of the economy and of society itself, but in doing this job in a very particular way for the capitalist economy women are guided by the State. This is not widely recognized.

To state so baldly that women have this particular 'job' in life may seem crude and over-simplified, although, as will later appear, Beveridge himself phrased it in terms no less crude; but it is difficult for us to perceive woman's role as a 'job' because of the sphere in which it takes place. That sphere is the family.

The institution of the family in modern, post-war society has been subjected to much sociological and psychological examination. During the past seven years it has also been a focus of controversy on the political Left, amongst feminists, socialists, and radicals of all kinds. It has come under attack; it has been defended. Often this debate, originally political, has taken on a highly moralistic flavour, and while it is true that political passions are, ultimately, moral passions, moralism about the family has all too often prevented a constructive analysis of this institution as it exists in our contemporary society. Yet it is not hard to understand why the subject should arouse passion; the same reason makes it hard to perceive woman's role within it

8

as a job, and the reason is that the family, for most people, is the only place where they give and receive affection. There, physical care is mediated by means of on-going emotional and physical relationships of the most intense kind; sexual and parental. Women in particular are reared almost from birth, certainly from early childhood, to conceive of happiness and emotional fulfilment in terms of their future relationship with husband and children. To many it therefore seems alien or even sacrilegious to discuss these relationships as jobs undertaken for the capitalist State. Nonetheless, such is the peculiar nature of the family. It plays what is in many ways a repressive role on behalf of the State, not only psychologically but also at the level of economic functioning, and yet at the same time offers the individual a unique opportunity for intimacy, comfort, and emotional support. In some ways, as Juliet Mitchell (1971) and Nigel Armistead (1974), among others, have pointed out, its values, stressing the mutual support of the group, are in conflict with the individualistic competitiveness of the wider modern society. This adds to its ambivalence – for many it is truly a 'prison of love'. And the Welfare State has always been closely connected with the development of the family and has acted to reinforce and support it in significant ways. This it has done by offering various forms of service, both in money and in kind, and also by means of forms of social control and ideology. Thus the Welfare State is not just a set of services, it is also a set of ideas about society, about the family, and – not least important – about women, who have a centrally important role within the family, as its linchpin.

To put it in a slightly different way, social policy is simply one aspect of the capitalist State, an acceptable face of capitalism, and social welfare policies amount to no less than the *State organization of domestic life.* Women encounter State repression within the very bosom of the family. This may seem paradoxical when the ideology of individualism and private property that has grown with capitalism has stressed the sanctity of family privacy. But in many ways the Welfare State, like the position of women, is full of paradox and contradiction.

One reason for the intense disagreements within the Left as to the nature of the family as an institution relates to the kind of socialism dominant in this country and Western Europe between 1945 and the late sixties when the student revolts, the Women's Movement, and the New Left generally, once more raised questions it had not been possible to raise for many years. These movements, the Women's Movement most strikingly, raised political and ideological questions, thereby challenging the then prevailing economism of the Left. Students began to question their own educational institutions instead of simply allying themselves to the workers in a mechanical way. Women began to question the structures that held them locked in sub-servience.

Nicos Poulantzas (1972) has commented on the comparative neglect amongst Marxists of the theory of the State and of political power. This he ascribes in part to economism. Econom-ism, a deviation towards the Right from orthodox Marxist theory and practice, reduces all other levels of social reality, the State included, to the economic, and therefore lays stress on political activity around wages and trades union struggle while neglecting ideology. This leads to a short-term, reformist per-spective.* Attitudes on the Left in the post-war period to the Beveridgean Welfare State offer a good example of economism in practice. Many socialists at that period accepted Beveridge as a step towards socialism, if not socialism itself, while as late as 1964 *A Socialist View of Social Work*, put out by social workers in the Socialist Medical Association, accepted a non-Marxist split between the emotional needs and the environmental needs of individuals, and repeated semi-psychoanalytical ideas about the emotional growth of the individual with little apparent under-standing of the structural and dynamic relationship of con-sciousness itself to environmental realities. One's very person-ality, outlook, feelings, and thoughts are formed to a large ex-tent by one's social environment, which includes one's class position and relationship to the economy. Applied to the Wel-fare State economism has meant in practice that traditional socialists have tended to misunderstand it, seeing it as a con-stellation of institutions that would be perfectly all right if we had more hospital beds, better schools with more teachers and less over-crowding, lower rents, higher sickness and unemploy-ment benefits, and decent pensions; an emphasis on the econ-omic aspects of the Welfare State coupled with an exclusion

* See note on page 187.

of – indeed a blindness to – its ideology. Marx himself said: 'Existence determines consciousness'. In practice economism has ignored consciousness and denied the relevance of emotions and relationships to Marxism, seeing them, in puritanical and conservative fashion as 'natural' and unproblematical, so that Peter Townsend (1958) for example, claiming to speak as a Socialist could nevertheless write:

> 'Traditionally Socialists have ignored the family or they have openly tried to weaken it – alleging nepotism and the restrictions placed upon individual families by family ties. Extreme attempts to create societies on a basis other than the family have failed dismally. It is significant that a Socialist usually addresses a colleague as "brother" and a Communist uses the term "comrade". The chief means of fulfilment in life is to be a member of, and reproduce a family. There is nothing to be gained by concealing this truth.'

This attitude accounts in part for the hostility within the Left towards the Women's Liberation Movement.

In his account of the capitalist state Poulantzas has drawn attention to its peculiar ambiguities, essentially elaborating on the passage in the *Communist Manifesto* (Marx and Engels 1970) (quoted at the front of this book) in which Marx and Engels described 'Bourgeois Socialism'. The capitalist State is a class State, yet the ideology of the bourgeois State is one that excludes class struggle, for: 'it presents itself as a state of the bourgeois class, implying that all the "people" are part of this class' (Poulantzas 1973). The Welfare State is one very important way in which a belief is fostered that our society is in fact 'classless', that 'we are all middle class now', or, as Anthony Crosland (1958) suggested, that we live in a 'post-capitalist' society, a society that has abolished the evils of capitalism without falling into the bottomless pit of 'totalitarianism'. As Victor George and Paul Wilding (1972a: 238, 240) put it:

> 'The dominance of the consensus model in thinking about social policy has meant that the Welfare State is seen as the result of the "general will" and that it is for the "public good" ... The Webbs spoke of the "capitalist domination of the mental environment" meaning the way in which nearly all our thinking about social and economic issues is shaped,

usually without us recognising the fact, by the particular nature of our economic system. Through it, certain sectional values and interests come to be seen and accepted as national interests.'

This is how most of us have been brought up; to see 'our' governmental system, civil service, law courts, police force, and social security as acting for all of us, for the 'nation' seen as a unitary and unified whole.

What is the Welfare State? The phrase is itself an aspect of the ideology to which it alludes, and the Welfare State is made up of both the welfare policies and the ideology in which they come wrapped. Writers commenting from within a traditional perspective have sometimes been quicker to see this than have socialists. Kenneth Boulding for example suggests that it is best to think of a spectrum ranging from economic policies at one end to social policies at the other, while beyond them, policies on delinquency, crime, and the police would eventually merge with defence policy and international relations and would pass beyond the bounds of what could reasonably be classed as social policy. Not content with this definition, however, Boulding goes on to add the ideological component:

'If there is one common thread that unites all aspects of social policy and distinguishes them from merely economic policy it is the thread of what has elsewhere been called the "integrative system" ... The institutions with which social policy is especially concerned, such as the school, family, church, or, at the other end, the public assistance court, prison or criminal gang all reflect degrees of integration and community. By and large it is an objective of social policy to build the identity of a person around some community with which he is associated ... Social policy is that which is centred in those institutions that create integration and discourage alienation.' (Boulding 1967:6)

This implies that social policy is an instrument whereby governments try to create a particular kind of society, and Boulding gives an illuminating example, minimum incomes policy. Social policies see to it that such provisions as exist – national insurance, supplementary benefit, family incomes supplement – are so distributed as to bring about a particular desired state of affairs. For example, a woman who cohabits with a man by that act forefeits her right to her own supplementary benefit. This ruling reflects a society in which women continue to be economically dependent upon men and a society in which this is convenient and also seems right and proper to many people – the traditional family relationships being seen very much as creating integration.

This does not mean that the Welfare State is a conscious conspiracy on the part of capitalism seen as a completely rational monolith. On the contrary, there are competing interests and factions within the dominant classes, as well as miscalculations and, at times, an anarchic absence of plan. Furthermore, the ideology of the 'general will' and the 'public good' does express a reality; that the State offers certain concessions to the economic interests of the dominated classes which may in fact be against the short term interests of those who wield power, but which do not endanger, and possibly do promote, their long term domination. Poulantzas (1973) argues that the Welfare State is an example of this kind of economic sacrifice – a little more of the wealth of our society is offered to all by means of welfare benefits, but there is no transfer of political power.

The State and State power remain repressive, although it is possible to distinguish between directly repressive aspects of the State and ideological institutions. This is not to say that institutions which purvey and transmit ideology are not repressive in a general sense, but they do not 'function by violence' (Althusser 1970) in the way that the repressive arm of the State does. Theirs is the sphere of psychological repression. Yet, schools, family, social services departments, also operate with the threat of ultimate violence at their disposal.

Think, for instance, of the difference between the police and social workers. 'Radical' criticisms of social workers have partly centred round the accusation that they are 'social policemen', or 'just the same as' the police. In fact, despite attempts by the police (especially policewomen) to emphasize their own social work role – as with the institution of the juvenile bureau – and in spite of the approximation of the social worker's role to that of the police in some of their more coercive duties, it is precisely the differences between the policeman's and the social worker's role that illustrates the difference between the directly repressive

State and the ideological repression of the State.

Ideological institutions ensure not simply the continuance of things as they are, but the acquiesence of the oppressed in their own economic and ideological oppression and exploitation. The exploration of this question – the search for an explanation of the reasons why workers, for the most part, need not be policed at the point of a gun – has turned out to be related to the position of women in a fundamental way. Ken Coates and Richard Silburn (1968) found in their study of a poor neighbourhood in Nottingham that the poor people they talked to either did not feel they should be rich or else conceived of an improvement in their income in incredibly circumscribed terms (£50 more per week was the largest sum mentioned, and those questioned seemed to have no real imaginative grasp of the economic gulf between themselves and the rich). Similarly one of the problems facing the Women's Movement has been that many women cannot really imagine a different kind of life for themselves. They can imagine perhaps getting more housekeeping money each week, or getting a nursery place for a child, but everything that they have ever experienced will have reinforced a view that there is no fundamental alternative, that marriage and children is right and proper for every woman. The shock of criticisms of this view from the Women's Movement has at times led to resentment and suspicion of Women's Liberation (although this has also been due to sensationalizing media coverage of the Movement). In seeking to understand why many women want things to remain as they are, feminists began to write about their own lives and the lives of other women, at first descriptively, later more analytically. And in exploring the day to day *work* of women in the home it was possible to make what amounted to a rediscovery of a Marxist concept: the reproduction of labour power, and the reproduction of the relations of production.

In order to continue, the capitalist mode of production must reproduce itself. Not only must the adult worker be enabled to present himself today, tomorrow, and every subsequent working day at the workplace; so must his children when their turn comes. The State plays its part in ensuring that these children not only learn the practical skills that will prepare them to become machine operatives, clerks, or managers, but also to learn

14

this 'in forms which ensure their subjection to the ruling ideology, or the mastery of its practice' (Althusser 1970: 128). In other words, the whole socialization and education process, at home and in the school, is of crucial importance in raising children who are both trained in particular ways to fit them for the various kinds of work necessary and available under capitalism, and trained to a belief in the naturalness and inevitability of this process. It is this process that the Welfare State is concerned to guide and promote, and in order to do this successfully it has had to develop a particular attitude towards women and the family.

Victorian and modern attitudes to women are closely linked with the whole development of the idea of childhood, which is of great significance in modern bourgeois society. Its extension and overvaluation has been part of the growth and development of capitalism itself. This was because the development of technology meant that many more children survived birth and babyhood, and the high mortality rates of earlier times were ended. The concept of the child-in-the-nuclear-family is central to the modern Welfare State; whilst alarm for the well-being of the children of the poor, in factories and workhouses, formed the take-off for early Victorian welfare provisions, as the new Inspectorate, with its blue books and reports, revealed to the horrified Victorians the dissolution of family life and the abandonment of children to vice and moral, if not political, subversion (these two then, as now, being linked in the ruling-class mind).

In the Middle Ages there was hardly a concept of 'child' at all and most babies died in infancy. Children who did survive were commonly sent away, from the age of about seven, to be trained and educated by strangers; they mixed freely with adults, and their discourse did not exclude discussion of sexual matters. Philippe Ariés (1973) suggests that during the seventeenth century a significant change took place, and the idea of the innocence of childhood won gradual acceptance. He connects this change with the rise of Puritanism, which brought with it also the beginnings of a belief in the importance of education, specifically moral training, for the child. The emergence of the school as a distinct social form indicates an increased interest amongst parents in their children's well-being, and Ariés stresses the importance of education and the school in creating a different and separate world for the child who had in former times been heedlessly allowed to mingle at his will with adults in all spheres of life, at work and play, eating and sleeping, at home and in the street. With the growth of the importance of the child goes a growth in the importance of the notion of family, and with this the importance attached to personal and familial privacy. Comfort, Ariés suggests, was born at this period, linked with, and a manifestation of, 'domesticity, privacy and isolation'. No longer did families eat and sleep in the same room; each room was reserved for a particular function. Comfort was also connected with hygiene. During the eighteenth century improvements in medicine and a greater understanding of the importance of hygiene led to increased life expectancy. Also at this time came the demographic revolution, and at the end of the century Malthus propounded his ideas on population increase. By the Victorian period the carelessness that went with the inevitability of death in childhood had entirely disappeared, indeed the Victorian obsession with death in childhood surely arose because while still rather common, it *was* no longer inevitable. Ariés points to the importance of the beginnings of discussion of birth control, and a changed attitude towards the numbers of children born once the idea of natural wastage became less relevant. Malthusian doctrines were influential from the end of the eighteenth century in the sense that they were discussed by economists and politicians as the problems of a rapidly increasing population began to cause alarm. The size of the bourgeois family did not begin to decline until the 1870s, however (Banks and Banks 1964), although methods of birth control were known and practised before that (Laslett 1965).

Theodore Zeldin (1973), using the work of David Hunt (1970) to modify that of Ariés, has suggested that there was conflict and confusion about child rearing practices well before the seventeenth century. He emphasizes particularly the restrained relations between mothers and their children: 'It was six months before Louis XIII's mother embraced him and his relations with her remained cold until his father died. Till then the mother belonged to the father. While their fathers were alive children could not get at their mothers' (Zeldin 1973:316).

Zeldin gives no other examples of this restraint between mothers and their children, but, if true, then it would imply that the rise and development of the ideal of Motherhood was an advance for woman in so far as it marked a progression away from her status merely as a chattel of her husband. It would also, of course, link with changing attitudes towards children. Here Zeldin notes a marked change during the course of the eighteenth century. Then for the first time the baby's and child's need for affection began to be stressed, along with the dangers of sexual over-stimulation.

Of central importance in the industrial revolution were the changes brought about in the lives of women and children. In the pre-industrial world of Britain work and home were not sharply separated as they became during the course of the industrial revolution and as they have remained since. Conflicting reconstructions (Perkin 1969) of family life prior to industrialization have been made, but it does seem clear that typically husband, wife, and children worked together and work shaded into the rest of life, as kinship shaded into community. In some ways the old order was highly restrictive. The notion of women and children as the property of the man remained. As late as the eighteenth century, Clarissa Harlowe, in Samuel Richardson's novel of that name, a daughter of a *nouveau riche* family, is required to marry an impoverished aristocrat, and is told she is lucky not to be physically beaten into submission when she refuses this man of her family's choice. Furthermore, the position of women reflected the general tone of society :

'In the small communities, the villages and tiny towns, of the old society ... the source of income itself, with the rest of the "life chances" of the individual, was controlled by a paternal landlord, employer or patron who regarded class attitudes as the insubordination of a dependent child. In a world of personal dependency any breach of the "great law of subordination", between master and servant, squire and villager, husband and wife, father and child, was a sort of petty treason, to be ruthlessly suppressed ... Literally so in the case of women who murdered, or were accessory to the murder of their husbands, who were burned at the stake for "petty treason".' (Perkin 1969:37)

Yet in other ways when work and family roles were less highly differentiated women in practice might have more freedom. The effect of economic and social change in the nineteenth century was to delineate women's roles more rigidly, and this meant that in many ways they were worse off than before. Changes were of three kinds.

There were changes in the conditions of work of women and children. Women had always worked. In a pre-industrial society of low productivity work was a family affair. Industrialization eventually drove women and children into the factories. Everywhere the development of capitalistic processes led sooner or later to an increasing division of labour, and, then women tended to be confined to certain occupations. Ivy Pinchbeck (1930) points out that already by the eighteenth century there were no women clothiers in any way comparable with the Wife of Bath and other independent fourteenth century businesswomen; and concludes that the apprenticeship system tended to exclude girls, who could always be usefully employed at home. On the farms women were gradually excluded from outdoor work and from the elaborate processes of dairy work, hitherto their exclusive province; accustomed to caring for the sick, they were excluded from the new opportunities for scientific medical training that arose out of the hospital movement of the second half of the eighteenth century; they were excluded from the business world as this gradually reorganized itself round the changing industrial scene, requiring new forms of financing and larger sums of capital, which meant that most women were necessarily unable to participate.

The factory system which substituted a family man's wages for a family wage was much hated at first, since, natural though the physical and social division between workplace and home has come to seem·to us, to the workers of those days it appeared entirely unnatural. Nor was it everywhere regarded as 'natural' that women should work outside the home at all, and in the factory districts men fought to get women out of factories rather than to unionize them within them. The disintegration of the family as a result of industrialization was, like industrialization itself, a gradual process, only completed in the 1820s and 1830s. At an earlier stage the traditional features of family work were retained even within the factory system, so that children often still worked for their fathers. But later the men began to be superseded altogether in the new factories, by women and children:

> 'Let us examine somewhat more closely the fact that machinery more and more supersedes the work of men. The human labour involved in both spinning and weaving, consists chiefly in piecing broken threads, as the machine does the rest. This work requires no muscular strength, but only flexibility of finger. Men are, therefore, not only not needed for it, but actually, by reason of the greater muscular development of the hand, less fit for it than women and children, and are, therefore, naturally almost superseded by them. Hence, the more the use of the arms, the expenditure of strength, can be transferred to steam or water power, the fewer men need be employed; and as women and children work more cheaply, and in these branches better than men, they take their place.' (Engels: 1973:179)

The involvement of working men in the agitation for the *Factory Acts* may, therefore, be interpreted as an attempt to restore the traditional family work arrangements and as a protest against the new, more differentiated work roles and family structure. In the 1840s factory agitation centred around the limitation of women's hours of work and around the education of children, and this reflects the importance of formal (State) education and the importance of the role of women in the socialization of children *in the home* which was one result of the industrial revolution (Smelser 1969). Influences that shaped the *Factory Acts* were of course more complex than this, and the work of Lord Shaftesbury, for example, represented in part the new evangelical puritanism with its repressive view of female sexuality. The degradation of the women who worked in the mines aroused horror not so much because of the degree of exploitation to which they are subjected but because the offence to morality and decency was so great (Hammond and Hammond 1969).

It is also important to remember that the *Factory Acts* extended the definition of a minor to include women. They gave legal sanction to the Victorian view that women simply were not responsible adults. Although women (and children) did of course continue to work outside the home, this began to cease being seen as 'natural' and the way was open to the modern extension of the whole concept of childhood, and the modern ambivalence towards the working mother. The question of women and children working was henceforth posed as a moral one.

There were advantages. Single women and widows especially (E. P. Thompson 1968) were freed from the humiliation of dependence on relations or parish relief and their status was raised, although on the other hand they became more dependent on employers and the labour market. A contemporary report stresses the progressive side of factory employment for women:

'One of the greatest advantages resulting from the progress of manufacturing industry and from severe manual labour being superseded by machinery is its tendency to raise the condition of women. Education only is wanting to place the women of Lancashire higher in the social scale than in any other part of the world. The great drawback to female happiness, among the middle and working classes is their complete dependence and almost helplessness in securing the means of subsistence. The want of other employment than the needle cheapens their labour in ordinary cases until it is almost valueless. In Lancashire profitable employment for females is abundant ... I believe it to be to the interest of the community that every young woman should have this in her power. She is not then driven into an early marriage by the necessity of seeking a home; and a consciousness of independence in being able to earn her own living, is favourable to the development of her best moral energies.' (Hickson 1840:44)

On the other hand factory work meant the emergence of the modern idea of woman's 'two roles' for the married woman, as Ellen Barlee observed in 1862:

'The dressmakers ... thrive upon such an occupied female population, for Lancashire lassies rarely make their own dresses. They can, however, pay well to have them done and it is therefore worthwhile for the dressmakers to study fashions and fits; so that on Sundays and holidays I was told it was quite surprising to see the elegant appearance these girls made ... On Saturday mills are closed at midday and the men and single women make real holiday. Then the town is all alive; it is quite a gala day; the men appearing in good broadcloth suits, and the girls as smart as wages can make them. The married women, who seem the slaves of Lancashire society, are obliged then, however, to set to work harder than ever. They have only this day to clean their houses, provide for the week, bake for the family, mend clothes, besides doing any washing that is not put out and attend the market to purchase the Sunday's dinner ... Then there is also washing the children and setting them to rights, always the Saturday night's business in every cottage – so that the poor mother seldom gets a rest ere the Sabbath dawns if indeed she is not up all night.' (Barlee 1863:25-7)

Moreover the dirt and overcrowding in the urban slums made the work of the housewife much harder; and all writers stress that the new life was worse for women than for men. One health inspector wrote:

' "Amidst these scenes of wretchedness, the lot of the female sex is much the hardest. The man, if as is usually the case, in employment, is taken away from the annoyances around his dwelling during the day, and is generally disposed to sleep soundly after his labour during the night; but the woman is obliged to remain constantly in the close court or neglected narrow alley where she lives, surrounded by all the evils adverted to; dirty children, domestic brawls, and drunken disputes meet her on every side and every hour. Under such circumstances, the appropriate employments of a tidy housewife in brushing, washing or cleaning, seem vain and useless efforts, and she abandons them." '
(Hammond and Hammond 1930:103-4)

Another inspector emphasized the valiant efforts these women continued to make:

' "It was often very affecting to see how resolutely they strove for decency and cleanliness amidst the most adverse circumstances; to see the floors of their houses and the steps washed clean, made white with the hearth-stone, when the first persons coming into the house must spoil their labours with the mud from the street, kept filthy by neglect of proper scavenging; to see their clothes washed and hung out to dry but befouled by soot from the neighbouring furnaces; and to see their children, attempted to be kept clean, but made dirty from the like causes." '

(Hammond and Hammond 1930 : 103)

As well as changes in the working lives of women, there were changes in their legal status. This linked with a third change, the development of bourgeois women into a leisure class playing an ideological rather than a directly economic role in their society. As the bourgeoisie expanded and became more prosperous, a part of the raised standard of living was leisure, and in particular the leisure of the wife or mother. Also, for the first time the woman as consumer became important, while the luxurious display with which she surrounded herself demonstrated her husband's success and wealth. At the same time her leisure depended on her working-class sisters, the flood of female labour that the industrial revolution had brought to the towns, to work the new machines or to be hired cheaply as domestic labour. With these changed conditions came a conscious, worked-up ideology of the Perfect Lady, the 'Angel in the House'. The idealized Wife/Mother was consciously perceived by writers and moralists of the period as providing an essential service for capitalism (Basch 1974) and the definition of woman as it was evolved by the Victorians was no mere flourish on the surface of their society; it was at the heart of Victorian capitalism. Woman provided the nest, the retreat, the temple, to which the bourgeois businessmen could return to rest from the harsh world of commerce. Thus Ruskin, perhaps most famous of all the apologists for woman's place, wrote:

'The woman's power is for rule, not for battle and her intellect is not for invention or recreation, but sweet ordering, arrangement and decision ... By her office and place, she is protected from all danger and temptation. The man ... must encounter all peril and trial; to him, therefore, must be the failure, the offence, the inevitable error; often he must be wounded, or subdued; often misled and *always* hardened. But he guards the woman from all this: within his house, as ruled by her, need enter no danger, no temptation, no cause of error or offence. This is the true nature of home – it is the place of Peace; the shelter not only from all injury, but from all terror, doubt and division.' (Ruskin 1865 : 144–45)

The married woman's physiological role as mother gave her also a special moral role. Yet it was full of contradictions. Her existence as a leisure object and luxury consumer conflicted with the work ethic so that a new emphasis had to be laid on the importance and complexity of ladylike domestic work. The early feminists were aware of this, and critical of it. Emily Davies, for instance, wrote:

' "Marriage is not a modern discovery, offering a hitherto untrodden field of action for feminine energy. The novelty is, that ... the old field has been invaded and taken possession of by machinery. The married ladies of former days, instead of sitting in drawing rooms, eating the bread of idleness, got through a vast amount of household business which their successors cannot possibly do, simply because it is not there to be done." ' (Banks and Banks 1964 : 49)

and Frances Power Cobbe in an essay that anticipates Simone de Beauvoir, pointed out how this can end by invading and distorting the whole feminine personality:

'The more womanly a woman is, the more she is sure to throw her personality over the home, and transform it, from a mere eating and sleeping place, or an upholsterer's showroom, into a sort of outermost garment of her soul; harmonised with all her nature as the robe and the flower in her hair are harmonised with her bodily beauty. The arrangement of her rooms, the light and shade, warmth and coolness, sweet odours, and soft and rich colours, are not like the devices of a well-trained servant or tradesman. They are the expression of the character of the woman ... A woman whose home does not bear to her this relation of nest to bird, calyx to flower, shell to mollusc, is in one or another imperfect condition. She is either not really mistress of her home; or being so, she is herself deficient in the womanly power of thoroughly imposing her personality upon her belongings.'
(Butler 1869 : 10–11)

There was also an extension of woman's Madonna role into the public sphere, and although it was generally considered undesirable for a 'lady' to work, she was encouraged to interest herself in the poor, to set her poor sisters a good example by performing good works. This was the origin of social work. To work for money, on the other hand, was to put herself beyond the pale of polite society, hence the ambiguous and pathetic position of governesses, who were neither servants nor yet of the family.

The development of middle-class women into a leisure class threw into more glaring relief the differences between their official, exalted status and their actual legal status as minors. A woman, once married, lost all rights over her own children, also over her own property, which became her husband's, and over any earnings she made subsequent to the marriage. It was only in the nineteenth century, when all the loopholes had been stopped up, that marriage actually became what it had always been intended to be, that is, indissoluble, but as the writers of the *Finer Report* (Vol II 1974:97) have pointed out:

> 'Theologically sound or not, a doctrine which to so large an extent delivered up a woman's property to her husband was not acceptable to the propertied classes. It became increasingly unacceptable as the leasehold grew in importance as a form of investment property, and fortunes were made in money, rather than through the ownership of land. This was because both money and leaseholds ranked in law as chattel interests over which ... the husband by contracting the marriage automatically gained absolute or near absolute dominion.'

Thus campaigns for change arose less from a sense of justice and equity than for material, economic reasons, and likewise the new morality of the Victorians also had a material basis:

> 'That "damned morality" which disturbed Lord Melbourne did not result from religious enthusiasm only. Differing provisions for the inheritance of family property were an important factor too. The sexual waywardness of the territorial aristocracy did not endanger the integrity or succession of estates which were regulated by primogeniture and entail. Countless children of the mist played happily in Whig and

Tory nurseries where they presented no threat to the property or interests of heirs. But middle class families handed their accumulating industrial wealth within a system of partible inheritance which demanded a more severe morality imposing higher standards upon women than upon men. An adulterous wife might be the means of planting a fraudulent claimant upon its property in the heart of the family; to avoid this ultimate catastrophe, middle class women were required to observe an inviolable rule of chastity.'

(*Finer Report* Vol II 1974:117)

It is important to remember that women themselves acquiesced in the myth of their own purity and asexuality. (Cristabel Pankhurst, for instance, was fanatical in her separatist belief in the superiority and purity of women, and the necessity for them to retreat, even if only for a time, from the degradation of relationships with men.)

Nor was the ideal of the Angel in the House confined to the bourgeoisie. It was also influential amongst those spokesmen for the working class who sought to change society. The Chartists did not after all demand the suffrage for women, but for men only; while their leader, William Lovett, hymned woman's role:

> *Her mission 'tis in youth's delightful spring*
> *Of gladsome life and ever flowering hopes*
> *With those persuasive powers which love inspires*
> *To calm our rugged and tumultous thoughts ...*
>
> *If she her household mission wisely fill*
> *Her home will be his refuge and his joy ...*
> *A household goddess worthy of all love*
> *In purity and smiles forever clothed ...*
>
> *The sexes' duties are so oft reversed*
> *Shame! in this flourishing and hopeful isle ...*
> *That here with power so vast mankind to bless*
> *Where gathered wealth might brighten every face*
> *Poor toiling woman from her home is driven*
> *And home becomes without her fostering care*
> *A place where misery scarcely rests its head ...*
> *Must wretched mothers call from sooty mines*
> *When scarcely clad like brutes in harness vile*

> *They daily drag their wretched lives away* ...
> *Shall* home *that cozy kind expressive word* ...
> *Shall this great altar of our English hearts*
> *That million arms have often nerved to save*
> *Crumble at last to rear great Mammon's shrine?*
> *Shall homes neglected send their blight abroad*
> *To taint with vice each mother's buds of hope?*
>
> (Lovett 1856)

From this poem we may understand more clearly why working class radicals mistakenly embraced the bourgeois ideal of the Angel in the House, the perfect Wife and Mother. It was part of their protest against the general conditions of work created by the industrial revolution. It is also one of the saddest and most persistent themes in the history of socialism, the adoption of a reactionary attitude to women as part of the demand for decent material conditions of life.

The irony of this ideal of womanhood was that many of those women who would most happily have embraced it were prevented from doing so. In the first place there was a surplus of women, largely within the middle class it was believed. Secondly, working-class women could hardly aspire to it, given the poverty and frightful housing conditions they had to endure. The records of the police courts showed that cruelty towards women was correlated with overcrowding, and the attitude of men towards their womenfolk was often brutal. John Stuart Mill and Harriet Taylor campaigned on this issue in the mid-nineteenth century. Dickens wrote in his novels of women who were beaten, and he also portrayed, in the person of David Copperfield's mother, the sufferings to which middle-class women might be subjected. In her case, physical brutality was reserved for her child, but her own mental sufferings caused her premature death. Later in the century, Frances Power Cobbe wrote a pamphlet, *Wife Torture in England* (1878), and this led to the passing of the *Matrimonial Causes Act* enabling working-class women to gain legal separations from their husbands.

In spite of the many social changes that have occurred in the past 120 years, the Victorian ideal of womanhood still influences us all today and is deeply embedded in the sophisticated ideology of the Welfare State. To this we now turn.

TWO

Ideology & welfare

Welfare policies are linked with, indeed part of, the elaboration of the State that has occurred as a part of the rise of industrial capitalism and its development into fully fledged monopoly capitalism (Hobsbawm 1968a). Reflecting the needs of capitalism as it developed it also responded to the demands of the organized working class. These two contradictory forces acting upon welfare legislation are themselves influenced or distorted by the ideological component always present, which has stamped the Welfare State with attitudes repressive both to women and to 'the poor'. The ideology of the Welfare State displays itself in the way in which welfare provision works in practice (an example would be the assumptions underlying the ways in which scarce nursery places are rationed, or the kind of housing allocated to one-parent families). It expresses itself above all in what is written about social work and social workers; the literature of social work *is* the ideology of welfare capitalism.

An important part of the ideology of welfare has been the whole way in which discussion of state intervention has tended to confuse it with socialism. A central paradox, indeed, of the Welfare State is the way in which it developed as a system of massive State intervention, a web of bureaucratic control with strands clinging to every niche and corner of society and of private life, out of a society in which the dominant ideology was of individualism. This paradox has been discussed in various ways, and for a long time the interpretation of A. V. Dicey, as put forward in *Lectures on the Relation between Law and Opinion in the Nineteenth Century*, published in 1905, dominated the debate. Dicey posed a simplistic distinction between Benthamite individualism, supposed to have been dominant from the period of the *1832 Reform Bill* until 1870, and the period of collectivism from then until 1900. Dicey's definition of individualism is not always consistent or clear (Burn 1964), although when he wrote of 'the wisdom of leaving everyone free to pursue his own courses of action, so long as he did not trench on the like liberty or the rights of his fellows' (Burn 1964) he was simply paraphrasing John Stuart Mill's famous definition and expressing the curious liberal view of individual freedom as essentially a form of isolation, ultimately setting one man against another and: ' "based on the separation of man from man. It is the right of this separation, the right of the limited individual ... the right of self interest ... It lets every man find in other men not the realisation but rather the limitation of his own freedom" ' (MacClellan 1968 : 178–9). That such a view is still dominant may be seen by reading any standard textbook on social casework. For example: 'Casework is characterised by its direct concern for the well-being of the individual ... from its inception it has stressed the value of the individual ... and the right of each man to live in his own unique way provided he does not impinge upon the rights of others' (Hollis 1964 : 7).

Debate around State intervention was certainly already oc-curring in the early Victorian period (Roberts 1960) as early welfare legislation – the *Factory Acts* and the *Poor Law* of 1834

– brought the beginnings of centralized State control of local activity. One feature of the growth of centralism was the corresponding growth of the inspectorate, of a bureaucracy. The *Poor Law*, which in turn led to increasing anxieties about public health, was only one expression of ruling class feeling about the condition of the people. There were hardly any Royal Commissions before that on the *Poor Law*, but between then and 1849 there were nearly one hundred. There were minor as well as major reforms important in consolidating the new key role of centralized administration : legislation on prisons, the mentally ill, and municipal corporations all expanded the bureaucracy and strengthened (however weak by modern standards they remained) the links between central and local government. Linked to the growth of the bureaucracy was the increasing domination of a scientific-rationalist approach towards the study of society, and a faith in the power of knowledge. Knowledge would reform the working class, socially and morally. This was another contradictory aspect of Victorian centralism – that it came into being in order to make the individual more self-sufficient, in order to promote successful individualism. A new centralized administration was being erected to remedy social abuses, so that from the beginning welfare and bureaucracy were closely intertwined. Moreover the remedy to the horrors of the 'condition of the people' was seen essentially in terms of saving the working class from their own barbarism and reconciling them to the bourgeois order. The gulf between the classes, seen as increasing rather than diminishing, the drunkenness, vice, and squalor of the industrial cities, the increasing crime rates, the lack of religion, and the lack of 'habits of industry', these were to be eradicated by education, sanitation, and the rationalization of the *Poor Law*. Poverty was to be fought with religious morality and hygiene. These early assumptions of welfarism have hardly changed in 130 years. In particular the growth of urbanism weakened the forms of social control of the old villages and the rise of the Welfare State has all along been closely connected with the control of undesirable forms of behaviour. The preservation of the family also became a focus of alarm in the early Victorian period. The sexual promiscuity found in the common lodging houses and tenement slums and courts filled the Victorians with horror, as did the condition of poor children. However, as yet these facts did not lead to a preoccupation, which would come later, with the conscious *State* support of the family. At this time the rationalism of the Inspectors led them more towards reform by promotion of correct intellectual attitudes in the minds of working-class people, and they were perhaps blind to the emotional forces that seemed all the same so threatening when manifested in the shape of riots and debauchery.

In tending to equate collectivism with socialism A. V. Dicey endorsed he did not originate, a confusion that has persisted ever since, for while all socialists are collectivists, not all collectivists are necessarily socialists (Marwick 1973). This confusion became an important part of the debate around State welfare at the end of the nineteenth century, partly because State intervention was in fact increasing. One form it could take was the 'gas and water' socialism of Joseph Chamberlain in Birmingham. Using the *Artisans' Dwelling Act* of 1875 he municipalized the public utilities and initiated slum clearance and an improvement scheme that did not, however, include housing to replace the slums demolished, although it did include free libraries and an art gallery.

Rather different was the socialism of the Fabians. They implicitly claimed to have laid the foundations of the modern Welfare State, and were always ardent advocates of State intervention. Sidney and Beatrice Webb wrote the *1909 Minority Report of the Royal Commission on the Poor Law*. This proposed the break up of the Poor Law and the division of its functions amongst specialist departments to deal with health, children, and so on, and it is sometimes assumed that because this did happen after 1945, the Webbs were responsible for it (Hobsbawm 1968b). The subsistence minimum income inaugurated by Beveridge did, amongst other things, reflect a belief in the importance of the prevention of destitution, disease, and idleness that harked back to the 1909 *Minority Report* and to the ideology of National Efficiency in general. But although prevention might be seen as a Fabian idea, the Webbs' attitude to welfare reform was more authoritarian than that of the Atlee government, they opposed the insurance principle upon which the British social security system has been built and believed in a mixture of coercion and moral reform to get the unemployed back to work. They did not believe in universal free social services, but felt that those who could should pay. Yet whatever their objective effect on the shape of welfare reform, the way in which they discussed it has influenced what we believe about it – Fabianism has contributed to the ideology of welfare, as well as developing and perpetuating the equation of welfare intervention with socialism. Yet in many ways the Fabian doctrine came closer to what would now be called State capitalism than to socialism, particularly in its insistence that the advent of socialism was likely to be as an administrative necessity rather than as the outcome of a process of class struggle. This was well understood at the time, and William Paul, a member of the Socialist Labour Party during the First World War, summed up the genuine socialist arguments against Fabianism in no uncertain terms:

'The most original and by far the cleverest section of the middle class intellectuals have agitated for the extension of municipal and state enterprise. Many of them have seen that the safest investment for the funds of the middle class have been in municipal loans ... This explains why it comes about that in large cities such as Glasgow the cars, gas, water etc. had been municipalised long before any labour men entered the Council.

The middle class activity on behalf of State enterprise or control is due to the fact that the future of competitive Capitalism shows little hope of the intellectual proletarians improving their lot. With the extension of the activities of the State new avenues of well paid official jobs are opened up. The candidates for these official posts have to pass examinations for which they have to be specially prepared ... The economic ideal of the intellectual wage earner is a National State controlling the industry of the country, in which each is rewarded according to a weird theory called the "test of ability". Thus just as the Capitalist uses *capital* as the test of remuneration, just as the wage labourer demands the social organisation and control of the products of *labour*, so the middle class intellectual desires *ability* to be the test of income ... The Theorists of the middle class who demand State and municipal enterprise have been grouped under the banner of the Fabians ... [who label] these bourgeois reforms as socialism ... The most influential political leaders of the British Labour Movement have been advocating State owner-ship for over twenty years as Socialism ... and until re-cently made no sympathetic attempt to understand the aims of the Socialism of the International Proletariat. Every ad-vance in municipalisation was heralded as Socialism in prac-tice ... [but] a close scrutiny of the various undertakings controlled by the State ... clearly demonstrates that instead of these making for economic freedom of labour, they tend to reinforce Capitalism and perpetuate class rule.'

(Paul 1917 : 179–80)

While the importance of Fabianism has probably been over-rated, that of Christian Socialism in shaping twentieth century welfare reform has tended to be underrated. Christian Socialism owed much to the thinking of T. H. Green (Richter 1964), an Oxford philosopher, who stressed the benign role of the State in his writings. For him, the State was not coercive, but defined, harmonized, and ultimately embodied the rights of each indi-vidual member of it. Such a philosophy made possible the vision of the reconstruction of national life by the re-creation of a sense of community, and was carried into practice by those of Green's disciples who founded the Settlement Movement in the East End of London. Almost all the architects of twentieth century welfare provision – Atlee and Beveridge for example – had settlement experience, and they carried into practice the Christian Socialist belief that in order to make a man good you must first give him the basic necessities of life. This point of view was kindlier and more humane than the more 'scientific' approach of the Fabians. Neither represented what a Marxist would mean by socialism, and Arnold Toynbee, for instance, explicitly rejected Marxism in his definition of Christian Socialism :

'"We differ from Tory Socialism in so far as we are in favour, not of paternal but of fraternal government, and we differ from continental socialism because we accept the prin-ciple of private property and repudiate confiscation and violence ... To a reluctant admission of the necessity of State

action, we join a burning belief in duty and a deep spiritual
ideal of life." '   (Richter 1964:286)

It was not surprising that there should be discussion amongst
politicians and philanthropists of State intervention during this
period of 'Social Imperialism'. It reflected and commented upon
a social world in which State intervention was in fact increasing. Indeed, State intervention in the welfare field ran alongside
State intervention in the economy, which slowly but surely
gained momentum. All-out State intervention in the economy
for the purpose of winning the First World War (Milward 1970)
did not continue in peace time, but the inter-war period saw
the process of the monopolization of capital continuing, as the
operations of capital were rationalized by the creation of car-
tels and trusts helped on by government intervention (e.g. the
amalgamation of the railways in 1921) rather than by outright
nationalization. The same period also saw the continuous increase and development of welfare provision (Gilbert 1970; Marshall 1965) and particularly of various forms of unemployment
'dole' schemes.

The hand-to-mouth and incoherent nature of the schemes
which limped alongside the *Poor Law* reflected the peculiar
nature of British society between the wars. Lloyd George, Winston Churchill, and William Beveridge had all been well aware
of the reforms introduced by Bismarck's authoritarian Imperialist administration in Germany before the First World War, and
some of the British welfare reforms initiated by these Liberal
leaders between 1906 and 1911 had been in conscious imitation
of Bismarck. Under the Nazis the German State evolved an
ideology of welfare that meshed closely in with the general
ideological and economic drive of the State. But Britain could
never be like Germany. Bismarck's reforms had been aimed
directly at undermining and counteracting the appeal of the
powerful Marxist Social Democratic Party of his time, and
there was no such corresponding party in Britain capable of
offering a coherent and worked-out socialist view of society that
would attract large numbers of working people, despite the
heightened militancy of the labour movement in the later years
of the Victorian period up until the First World War. On the
other hand, the strength of the trades unions in Germany had

never equalled their position in Britain. Here, their strength was due precisely to their reformism, and after the collapse of the General Strike the incorporation of the TUC leadership into the power structure of British society continued (Hobsbawm 1968b; Hutt 1938; Foot 1973). So, even at a time of economic crisis the conflicting forces that have stamped the British Welfare State were clearly in operation: the persistence of economic liberalism which meant that in spite of continuing monopolization economic intervention by the government could never be wholehearted; the reformist strength of the labour movement, which damped down conflict by its acceptance of piecemeal legislation and was essentially without a worked-out analysis; and the belief even amongst feminists in the preservation of women's special role. The thrust of feminism wavered between the wars, partly because it was believed that with the vote women had achieved emancipation. The feminist organizations continued to be orientated towards Parliamentary reform, although now of a rather piecemeal kind, and although Sylvia Pankhurst and Eleanor Rathbone amongst others, paid a good deal of attention to the inadequacies of welfare provision for women, especially mothers, there was little analysis of women's Motherhood role. On the contrary, in practice, although in intention it was more complex, Eleanor Rathbone's campaign for the endowment of motherhood (a form of state allowance or salary for childcare in some ways akin to our family allowances) reinforced the belief in women's essential difference from men. Finally, the suspicions of welfare reforms among the working people for whom they were intended acted as a further brake both on the development of a coherent bourgeois ideology of welfare and on the development of socialist analysis.

After the Second World War the process of nationalization initiated by the Labour Government confirmed and accelerated the trend towards monopolization rather than steering the country in any sense towards a form of socialism. From then until recently, high employment policies were followed for political rather than economic reasons, because a repetition of unemployment on the scale of the thirties would not again, it was believed, be tolerated (Gough 1975; Devine 1974. For a critique of Gough's position, see Fine and Harris (1976 a and b). The continued development first of short term, later of long term capitalist planning of the economy both here and in other countries was an attempt (Warren 1972) to deal with the economic consequences of high employment policies. High employment and the Welfare State were part of the post-war settlement, the concessions made in return for 'social peace' and general union support of government policies that were often far from progressive. But this attempt to resolve the problems of the capitalist economy has itself created a new set of difficulties, which we experience today in the form of high unemployment coupled with inflation and the erosion of the welfare system that was created to both sweeten and strengthen capitalism.

The period since the Second World War is marked off from what went before by an intensification of state interest in family life and in the child. The earlier periods had given expression through social policy to an interest above all in the maintenance of the adult worker. Social Imperialism at the turn of the century inaugurated a progressively increasing interest in motherhood and the working-class family, but this interest could not flower until the establishment, with Beveridge, of a subsistence minimum income, however meagre. Similarly, feminism was under attack in the thirties, but it was not until the fifties that the ideological oppression of women became fully refined, along with the development of consensus politics. This also had an influence on the way in which welfare provision was perceived after the Second World War.

Dicey's interpretation of welfare provision was not seriously challenged until the 1940s. Then, in the context of the defence of Attlee's Welfare State, an alternative view was put forward which sought to explain its arrival in terms of its necessity. This functionalist view stressed the practical necessity of social policy as more than : 'mere sweeteners of the harsh rigours of a system of individualist compulsions. They represent social provision against waste of life and resources and against social inefficiency – not concessions' (Goldthorpe 1964 : 49), and H. L. Beales (1952) has emphasized the importance of State action in offsetting the uncertainty, insecurity, and social waste brought about by the *laissez-faire* of the early industrial revolution. E. H. Carr stressed the role of State intervention in preventing the escalation of class antagonisms into open rebellion and the disruption of the social order. There clearly is a sense in which state welfare legislation, as we know it, was a response to the changing conditions brought about by industrialization and urbanization in the early nineteenth century and thereafter; and the functionalist interpretation is still the dominant one today. Maurice Bruce, for example, defines his subject matter as follows:

'If then we seek to understand the Welfare State, we had best take it for what it is, the sum of efforts over many years to remedy the practical social difficulties and evils of a modern system of economic organisation which grew with but little regard for the majority of those who became involved in it ... The origins of many of the social problems which have had to be tackled are to be found in the conditions under which modern industry arose. To that extent the Welfare State is the practical British answer to the practical problems of industrial development and mass society which, though Britain was the pioneer, every people in the world now has to face.'   (Bruce 1968 : 1)

Yet this view is too simple for it ignores the ideology of the Welfare State and certainly cannot explain why that ideology has reinforced women's role in the way it has, nor why maintenance of the family has played so important a part.

I have suggested that the ideology of the Welfare State is best expressed today in the literature of social work. This literature is not – or certainly not always – overtly reactionary or conservative; rather it fetishizes change and innovation, as happens also in the production process where 'new models' constantly replace old. (Yet the 'new models' are always essentially the same as the old, Pincus and Minahan's book (1973) is an especially delicious example of old wine in new bottles, with a new jargon to describe the old activities). The latest word for social workers is indeed 'change-agent'. Just as modern capitalism and social democracy constantly attempt to incorporate revolutionary potential and to transform the truly progressive into a new prop for capitalism (the lip service paid to workers' control in the shape of worker directors would be one example), so social work is ever fetishizing some new *method* of work in order to evade the crucial issue of what its *function* is. When traditional psychotherapy, counselling, and social casework come under attack, or fail to damp down conflict, 'family sculpting', crisis intervention, and systems theory are feverishly brought into play. To state this is not to say that casework and counselling can never be helpful; on the contrary human beings commonly seek to discuss their feelings and problems and what is peculiar about our society is rather the way in which an expertise of talking to people about their difficulties has been developed from one particular model, the medical. What is oppressive about both new and old social work methods has been the persistent belief that the 'clients' for whom they are intended are inarticulate and express their emotions only in an impoverished way (MacBroom 1970). (Social workers are especially fond of the work of Basil Bernstein (1973) and interpret it to mean just this.)

Even more confusedly, alongside the traditional liberalism of social casework a bourgeois-radical ideology has grown up, sometimes incorporating ideas vaguely derived from Marx, although often misrepresenting Marxism (Holman 1973), more often derived from sociological theories of pluralism, labelling, and the like. But notions of client participation are no less mystifying than the efforts of former generations of philanthropists to make the poor independent and self-respecting; the development of community work and community action (Marris and Rein 1970) as an enterprise of the State to recuperate and contain local grass roots organization is still a form of containment even if it comes wrapped in radical rhetoric.

If radicalism misunderstands the rhetoric of 'change' from one angle, I have already suggested that, especially since the Second World War, traditional socialists have had an economistic analysis that has also failed to come to grips with the ambiguities of welfare. Thus, writers either assumed that the Welfare State was simply the fruit of mass demands and heroic struggle on the part of the working class, or saw it as a capitalist conspiracy to pacify the workers. Neither view confronts the ambivalence inherent in welfare provision, which reflects a deep contradiction of capitalism – a contradiction 'which enhance(s) human welfare and negate(s) it within the same process' (Leonard 1973:43).

It is not perhaps surprising that socialists have found it difficult to come to grips with this problem since this reflects the fragmentary nature of Marx's own writings on the subject (Mishra 1975), although he carried out an exhaustive study of factory legislation. Thus he can both understand the 'immense physical, moral and intellectual benefits' accruing to the workers from the *Factory Acts*, while at the same time he sees their purpose in restraining the worst excesses of capitalism, and also their functional purpose for the developing capitalist process:

' "Factory legislation, the first methodical and purposive reaction of society upon the uncontrolled and spontaneous development of its process of production is ... a no less inevitable product of large scale industry than are cotton yarn, self actors and the electric telegraph." '   (Mishra 1975:295)

At the same time Marx was clear that social needs would remain and would still need to be met under socialism:

'There remains the other part of the total product, designed to serve as means of consumption.
But before this is distrbuted to individuals the following further deductions must be made:
Firstly: the general costs of all administration not directly appertaining to production.
This part will, from the outset, be very significantly limited in comparison with the present society. It will diminish commensurately with the development of the new society.
Secondly: the amount set aside for needs communally satisfied, such as schools, health services, etc.
This part will, from the outset, be significantly greater than in the present society. It will grow commensurately with the development of the new society.
Thirdly: a fund for people unable to work, etc., in short, for what today comes under so-called official poor relief.'
(Marx and Engels 1970:318)

Marxists writing on welfare appear to have stressed one or other aspect of what Marx suggests only schematically and have not unnaturally fitted it to their own view. Thus Marxists tainted with economism have ignored ideology. On the other hand, libertarian attempts to come to grips with the nature of the Welfare State (notably the Claimants' Unions) have understood much better the repressive aspects of State provision, but have tended to fall into a conspiracy theory, and even to deny the need for State social provision at all. (For example, discussions of women's health within the Women's Movement have, at times, involved what almost amounts to a rejection of state medicine with a stress on nature cures, childbirth at home, and so on. But while it is right to be critical and suspicious of the drug industry, unnecessary induction of labour, and many other features of modern medical practice, the point surely is to use technology for our own benefit rather than rejecting it outright.)

Welfare provision, similar in some ways to the modern trades union movement, is an essential part of modern capitalism, and yet, although reformist, creates new economic and political problems for social democracy. It simultaneously tries both to keep us happy and to keep us down, and is part of the tight-rope act (Gough 1975) continually having to be performed by bourgeois democratic governments in their attempts to balance working-class demands and the reproduction of capital. It should also be said that however ambivalent the nature of welfare provision under capitalism, nevertheless an inadequate or punitive social security minimum is preferable to no minimum at all. It is certainly an important part of the class struggle to resist cuts in welfare and to agitate for more, particularly in a period of crisis when those in power will have little room for manoeuvre. Yet the earlier history of the Welfare State is characterized by a persistent thread of working-class hostility for State provision which has never been given status or even recognition in official histories of the subject.

Finally, the meaning of the Welfare State to women, who confront it daily, has been consistently ignored. I hope to make good that extraordinary, yet extraordinarily predictable omission, and to show that an analysis of the position of women is not marginal but central to a true understanding of the nature of the Welfare State. The ideology of the Welfare State has changed. In its beginnings, greater emphasis was placed on the immediate reproduction of the worker. Malthusian ideas meant that the dangers of over-population were stressed, rather than care for children already born. The main preoccupation was with the work ethic. Increasingly, and especially since 1945, the main emphasis has been on the reproduction of labour power in terms of children, the next generation. First and foremost today the Welfare State means the State controlling the way in which the woman does her job in the home of servicing the worker and bringing up their children. These constraints upon the way in which she does her job are less obvious than the demands of the assembly line, the rules and regulations of factory or shop work, but are for that very reason the more mystifying and insidious. This connection between the State and women's lives appears to have been largely forgotten or shelved for many years. An understanding of it is not new, however. In 1906 Beatrice Webb wrote to Millicent Garrett Fawcett to explain why, having previously been opposed to the Women's Suffrage Movement, she had now decided to support it:

'My objection was based principally on my disbelief in the validity of any "abstract rights" ... I prefer to regard life as a series of obligations ... I could not see that women are under any particular obligation to take part in the conduct of Government ... I thought that women might well be content to leave the rough and tumble of party politics to their mankind, with the object of concentrating all their own energies on what seemed to me their peculiar social obligations, the bearing of children, the advancement of learning, and the handing on from generation to generation of an appreciation of the spiritual life.

Such a division of labour between men and women is however only practicable if there is among both sections alike a continuous feeling of consent to what is being done by Government as their common agent. This consciousness of consent can hardly avoid being upset if the work of Government comes actively to overlap the particular obligations of an excluded class ... The rearing of children, the advancement of learning and the promotion of the spiritual – which I regard as the particular obligations of women – are, it is clear, more and more becoming the main preoccupations of the community as a whole. The legislatives of this century are in one country after another increasingly devoting themselves to these subjects. Whilst I rejoice in much of this new development of politics, I think it adequately accounts for the increasing restiveness of women. They are in my opinion rapidly losing their consciousness of consent in the work of Government and are even feeling a positive obligation to take part in directing this new activity. This is in my view, not a claim to rights nor an abandonment of women's particular obligations, but a desire more effectively to fulfil their functions by sharing the control of State Action in these Directions.'   (Webb 1926:362–63)

Neither feminist nor socialist, this passage nonetheless lays a finger on a central connection of modern life; that the development of welfare legislation is of intimate importance to women, and not simply of personal, but of political importance as well. The Six Demands of the Women's Liberation Movement implicitly recognize the centrality of state welfare care. They are: free abortion and contraception on demand; twenty-four hour nursery care; equality of education and job opportunity; legal and financial independence; a demand for recognition of the authenticity of lesbianism and the autonomy of women's sexuality; and equal pay.

For femininity the Women's Movement substitutes feminism. The feminist 'client' of the welfare services (although unlikely to call herself a feminist) is aware, as is the feminist social worker, of her position in the world and in relation to the State (indeed the instinctive gut reaction of clients to 'the Welfare' shows a correct understanding of its role). She is the client who is labelled 'anti-authoritarian', 'aggressive', 'problem mother', or 'castrating', and she has taken the first step towards taking control of her life by challenging the State's definition of her.

While the Women's Movement has spawned new ideas and refashioned old ones, its struggles have often seemed unanchored, cut off from many groups of women, from whole areas of working-class struggle, from the Left. Its continuing vitality has often come from sporadic activism and agitational propaganda only vaguely aimed, so that some of the writings of the Movement seem like a series of notes in bottles cast on the waves in the hope that someone – anyone – will eventually get the message. It is a tribute to the relevance of the ideas that so many women have in fact got the message.

The book is written particularly for the women (and men)

who work for the State, and for the women, housewives, mothers, and workers, who are subjected to its sexist ideology. It is intended as an exposure of that ideology. It is also a call to fight it.

THREE

Women, social welfare, & social work in Victorian society

In Victorian society women were, for the first time, valuable *because* they did not work. It was her status as a *non* worker that gave woman as Wife and Mother a very special ideological role. The single woman was society's reject, for celibacy was not highly valued (so that the attempts within the Church of England to start religious orders for women could be seen as radical (Deacon and Hill 1972)) while the fallen woman's lot was to be completely outcast (Basch 1974). Yet work had to be found for the army of surplus middle-class spinsters and to them fell the task of teaching their impoverished married sisters how to be better wives and mothers. So grew up a paradoxical situation that still marks social work today; whereby middle-class women with no direct experience of marriage and motherhood themselves took on the social task of teaching marriage and motherhood to working-class women who were widely believed to be ignorant and lacking when it came to their domestic tasks.

Bitter controversy raged around the subject of working wives and mothers. Lord Shaftesbury based his arguments for factory legislation on the disintegration of family life brought about by industrialization. Engels followed a contemporary writer, Peter Gaskell (1833) in describing how the new organization of work actually made the care of children impossible:

> 'We find ... the work of women up to the hour of confinement, incapacity as housekeepers, neglect of home and children, indifference or actual dislike to family life, and demoralisation; further, the crowding out of men from employment, the constant improvement of machinery, early emancipation of children, husbands supported by their wives and children ...'   (Engels 1973 : 236)

These critics probably exaggerated both the numbers of married women at work and the evils attendant upon this social fact (Hewitt 1958), but in any case various arguments against working mothers were widely current amongst the Victorians. For women to work was thought to cause early marriage, to encourage men to stay at home instead of themselves seeking work; yet, paradoxically, to prevent women from seeing after their homes properly and thereby driving men to the pub; to encourage also vice and immorality at the workplace. Margaret Hewitt (1958) in a study, primarily of the Lancashire textile districts, demonstrates that all the arguments used were based on insufficient and inconclusive evidence. For instance it is clear that working-class sexual morality in the nineteenth century never approximated to the ideals of the bourgeoisie. Peter Gaskell commenting on this quoted the Poor Law Commissioners:

> ' "It may safely be affirmed that the virtue of female chastity does not exist among the lower orders of England, except to a certain extent among the domestic female servants who know that they hold their position by that tenure and are more prudent in consequence." ' (Gaskell 1833 : 102)

while towards the end of the century Charles Allen Clarke observed: 'Though there is a good deal of sexual intercourse between young persons, this is not promiscuous, but between courting couples before marriage' (Clarke 1913). Flora Thompson (1973) described similarly the customs of the rural labourers in the 1880s and 1890s in Northamptonshire and Oxfordshire. Yet Shaftesbury's outraged cry: ' "Domestic life and domestic discipline must soon be at an end; society will consist of individuals no longer grouped in families; so early is the separation of husband and wife, of parents and children" ' (Hewitt 1958:10), expressed, if not the reality, the ideology of what people *believed* was happening, and that Victorians believed it had important effects on welfare legislation and the attitudes still today embodied in that legislation.

The Victorians were right in one way; there does seem to have been a clear connection between working mothers and infant mortality. Mothers of small children who went out to work whether it was in the factories or the fields, were seldom able to have their babies with them all day to suckle them, and so were forced to leave them in the care either of little girls aged as young as seven years, or of old women, 'day nurses' (i.e. baby minders), who did the thing for profit, often combining this with the trade of washerwoman. Victorian knowledge of baby care was rudimentary and the babies were usually fed on 'pap' which was bread softened and mashed in warm water and treacle or sugar. The nutritional properties of milk were not understood; in any case it was far too expensive for most working people, and also it was likely to be infected with tuberculosis germs. The babies were often given laudanum and other opiates too, to keep them quiet. Again, the dangers of these drugs were not popularly understood (and indeed the taking of laudanum was quite common amongst middle-class married women – yesterday's Valium; Jane Carlyle, for example, was addicted to it at one period in her life). Not surprisingly infant mortality was high, and this caused widespread alarm. Nevertheless, it was at first held that the State should not intervene. As late as 1874, Whately Cooks Taylor, addressing the National Association for the Promotion of Social Science could assert:

' "I would far rather see even a higher rate of infant mortality prevailing than has ever yet been proved against the factory districts or elsewhere . . . than intrude one iota further

on the sanctity of the domestic hearth and the decent seclu-
sion of private life ..."'   (Hewitt 1958:160)

Day nurseries were one possible solution to the problem. It
was at first thought that employers should provide these, since
they were held as much to blame for the situation as the
mothers themselves. But in the end it was charitable voluntary
effort that tried to provide day care for infants. The first day
nursery had been established in France in the early 1840s. By
1867 there were eighteen creches in Paris, ten in the suburbs and
four hundred in the provinces. In March 1850 the first voluntary nursery was opened in this country, in Marylebone, by a
group of women who had been inspired by the French example.

For a time nurseries were supported, especially by social
workers and doctors, as the solution to the problem. It was
noted that the Peabody Trust made special provision on its
estates for the infants of mothers amongst their tenants who
had to go out to work and the *Lancet* (see Hewitt 1958) thought
they offered a convenient outlet for the energies of women
'who now besiege the portals of our profession' (i.e. the medical
profession). Yet these nurseries, like so much official welfare provision whether furnished by the State or by voluntary effort
acting in the State's interest, were not overwhelmingly popular
with mothers. Perhaps because they required applicants to
answer searching questions about their morals and financial
situation, or because (as was the case in the Potteries) the
mothers hesitated to take money out of the hands of the old
women they had been accustomed to have care for their children. There was a preference, found over and over again, for the
provision of known and trusted neighbours, rather than for
official arrangements.

Towards the end of the century different remedies were
suggested, and some were tried. Again, this was in imitation of
experiments on the Continent. One factory owner at Mulhouse
had instituted a rudimentary insurance fund that enabled working mothers to take six weeks paid leave after the birth of a
baby. By 1906 Miss Squires, the Factory Inspectress, was saying:

' "Disastrous as are the consequences in so many instances
of the early return to work, one can neither be surprised nor

46

blame the mothers who take the risk of them rather than accept what seems to them the only alternative. Insurance of some kind against this recurring event seems a necessary adjunct to the enforcement of the law." ' (Hewitt 1958 : 180)

In Bismarck's Germany such a scheme had already been introduced, but not until 1911 was a similar first attempt made to insure maternity leave for working mothers in this country.

The law to which the woman factory inspector referred was another attempt to prevent mothers from returning to work too early; an Act of 1891 made it illegal for any employer to employ a woman within four weeks of her confinement. This provision was widely evaded, and indeed could not be enforced since women could conceal the exact date of their confinement; and usually they had to go back to work as early as possible if they had no man to provide for them, or if, as was equally common, their husband's wages were insufficient to keep the family from starvation. The unrealism of the law was attacked by feminists: Miss Ada Heather Bigg, Secretary of the Women's Employment Association, saw in the clause yet another attempt on the part of male trades unionists to drive women out of the labour market, and Elizabeth Garrett Anderson appears to have objected to its authoritarian nature.

On the one hand, then, there was a widespread belief in the inadequacies of the working-class woman as a housewife and mother; on the other the middle-class spinsters. There was also a widespread belief in the gulf between rich and poor, which was thought to be widening dangerously, and yet at the same time there was a consciousness of the sufferings of the masses, of which Victorian philanthropy was the expression. Modern social work has grown out of this coincidence of circumstances and the social worker's role was clearly from the first to re-create the Victorian family and improve the performance of the working-class mother.

As early as 1844 a Society for Improving the Condition of the Labouring Classes had been formed, with Lord Shaftesbury as its chairman. In the early 1850s Frederick Denison Maurice and the Christian Socialists were active, and in 1851 they began to found associations for co-operative production, which, they hoped, would give the workers a fair share of the profits of their labour. Aware of the problem of the surplus woman, and especially the surplus 'lady' they also founded a Ladies Co-operative Guild. Octavia Hill's mother was made manager of this Guild, and thus was Octavia Hill herself first involved in the sufferings of the poor.

Octavia Hill is an important figure in the development of social welfare. She brought forward to the turn of the century ideas in many ways characteristic of an earlier period, and her contribution to the ideology of social work – her emphasis on individualism and example – and her stress on the importance of training still influence it today (Moberley Bell 1942). Her work with the poor started when she began to teach classes for working women. She initiated a weekly meeting for women from the classes, where they learnt to make clothes for their children. She in her turn learnt from them of their atrocious living conditions and, with the support of Ruskin, founded a model lodgings house, the first of a number of such schemes. Her aim was to keep her slum properties clean and decent by enlisting the co-operation of her tenants not merely in keeping up to date with their rent but also in improving their condition of life. A family was started in one room; when they had proved they could live decently in this, they were offered the opportunity to expand into a second room. In this scheme great stress was laid on the importance of her personal relationship with her individual tenants. In a generous but clear sighted appreciation of her, Henrietta Barnett, with the kindlier perceptions of Christian Socialism, observed:

'She was strong-willed – some thought self-willed – but the strong will was never used for self. She was impatient in little things, persistent with long suffering in big ones; often dictatorial in manner but humble to self-effacement before those she loved or admired. She had high standards for everyone, for herself ruthlessly exalted ones, and she dealt out disapprobation and often scorn to those who fell below her standards for them, but she somewhat erred in sympathy by urging them to attain her standards for them, instead of their own for themselves ... I thought that her demands for the surroundings of the tenants were not high enough. She expected the degraded people to live in disreputable conditions until they had proved themselves worthy of better ones, whereas it can be argued that for most folk decent environment is essential to the promotion of decent life.'

(Barnett 1918 : 30)

She began her housing work in 1864. During the later 1860s alarm as to the condition of the London poor was already increasing amongst the wealthy. The geographical desertion by the rich of the poorer parts of the metropolis reinforced a belief that this severance of rich from poor was creating a dangerous social vacuum. To allay their fears many of the rich gave charity indiscriminately; but this also caused alarm, for charity in Victorian society could no longer perform its original purpose.

The stability of a static, medieval society had originally been reinforced by the paternalistic relationship between masters and peasantry. The rich man enjoyed his privileges, yet these also bestowed certain obligations upon him. He had a social duty to give, out of charity, to the poor and to provide for them when they were in distress, as his children; charitable works were also one way of giving thanks and worship to God. A third aspect of this relationship was that it served as a means of social control; in order to receive, the poor had to behave acceptably and with due deference. All this meant that charity was far from impersonal; it represented a complex web of social relations. By the nineteenth century this relationship had been completely swept away and charity had become a free handout. Because the nature of unemployment was not generally understood, many thought that charity actually caused pauperism, and must be controlled and regulated. In 1869 therefore the Charity Organisation Society (COS) was formed, again with the backing of Ruskin, and Octavia Hill became one of its first district organizers (in Marylebone).

The COS in its work of organizing and distributing charitable funds in order that these should henceforth go only to the 'deserving', developed the method of interviewing and recording that has become known as casework. It is important to remember that by 'deserving' the COS did not mean simply in terms of moral worth; they were also determined that money should not go to families as a kind of dole, but that it should be used where it could offer them the means of future self-help and self-sufficiency, so that its records are full of examples of widows being given sewing machines or the wherewithal to set themselves up as washerwomen. The personal relationship between the family to be helped and the COS visitor therefore became important since continued supervision, encouragement, and support became necessary when this kind of independence was the desired goal.

Social workers who have written on the subject have usually tried to separate the charity-regulation aspects of COS activity from the method the Society evolved to achieve its end – case-work. Kathleen Woodroofe (1962) for example concedes that the values of the COS were riddled with 'galling class-conscious-ness' but stresses the value of the casework method, which saw each applicant 'as an individual'. (Casework literature has always embodied the curious assumption that we do not usually do this.) She admits that:

'As a social sedative [the COS] served to damp down social discontent by stressing the duties which the rich owed the poor (a "sense of citizenship" as C. S. Loch called it), while denying the fact that the poor had the social rights of a citizen. By making its concessions to the alleviation of poverty, it helped, not only to recreate that "sense of mem-bership in social life" on which Loch set such store and which had been lost in the scrambling world of industrial-ism, but to eliminate the danger of social revolution.'

(Woodroofe 1962 : 50)

Yet she perceives another aspect of the work of the COS as admirable – its task as 'social regenerator', viewing the aim of the Victorian caseworker to cure the 'moral degeneration' of the pauper as a task to be applauded:

'In pursuing this aim the nineteenth century social worker ... evolved many principles which still form an essential part of the modern theory and practice of social casework ... (She learnt) how to ferret out, beneath the sur-face of dependence, apathy and hopelessness, some elements of character and will-power which could be utilised to bring the poor back to be self-respecting members of society.'

(Woodroofe 1962 : 51)

Even today, many well-meaning social workers find it hard to see what is wrong with such an aim, so imbued with the social work ideology that they fail to appreciate the assumptions that lie behind this message – that working-class people have weakness of character, a certain inadequacy and spinelessness, which only the assistance of their betters can help them overcome. But Gareth Stedman Jones on the other hand points out that it really is not possible thus to separate philosophy from method :

'The elaborate methods of investigation and classification devised by the COS were an attempt to reintroduce the element of obligation into the gift in districts where a small number of mainly non-resident rich were confronted with a vast and anonymous mass of poor applicants.'

(Stedman Jones 1971 : 257)

In other words, it was a way to make these applicants grateful and well-behaved, or of trying to.

In 1875 C. S. Loch was appointed Secretary of the COS, a post he retained until 1913. He was a fervent exponent of self-reliance and thrift, and it is important to remember that individualism meant in practice an emphasis on the self-reliance of the family; the individual was seen as a man, a wage earner with a responsibility for his family as well as for himself. Family obligations were the cornerstone of Loch's philosophy.

Helen Bosanquet, another pioneer social worker, also believed that State assistance and intervention were wrong because they were impersonal. Opposing State pension schemes, for example, she wrote: 'The COS have always been opposed to ... all plans for granting a stereotyped form of relief to large numbers of persons whose needs are very varying and only capable of being met by individual attention' (Bosanquet 1973 : 295). The organization of charity did not in fact act as a 'social sedative' in the straightforward way Kathleen Woodroofe suggests. During the later years of the nineteenth century there was a continued and intensified fear of the revolutionary menace of the poor. Octavia Hill's housing schemes could not solve, as had once been optimistically hoped, the problem of London's casual poor. Economic depression, unemployment, the chronic problem of urban housing that industrialism had created (and has never been able to solve), and several exceptionally hard winters brought matters to a crisis in London with the Trafalgar Square riots early in 1886. This came only three years after the publication of Andrew Mearns's *The Bitter Cry of Outcast London* (1883), one of a whole series of journalistic and often sensationalized exposures of the condition of the people. There began to be a new awareness that poverty was not invariably the fault of the poor themselves. The 'New Philanthrophy' also recognized that, now they had been granted the vote, working men had the power to alter the conditions under which they lived, and accordingly attempts to influence and guide the working masses took on new forms, notably that of the Settlement Movement (Stedman Jones 1971; Simon 1965) which represented the enactment of a new and more whole-hearted effort to improve the poor by example.

Louisa Twining was one of a number of pioneer women social workers who – more than Octavia Hill had done – stressed the particular role of women. Their work arose initially as a result of the criticisms of the *Poor Law* that had always been voiced (Pashley 1855). Louisa Twining, daughter of a London vicar, took up workhouse visiting in the course of helping her father just at the time when this type of good work, on a purely voluntary basis, was beginning to be accepted as a suitable task for ladies: 'In 1855, a volume of "Practical Letters to Ladies" was published, containing one by the Rev. J. S. Brewer on "Workhouse Visiting", which proved that the matter was beginning to be recognised as a duty' (Twining 1880:4), she wrote later, although visiting or indeed any interference from women met with much resistance from Boards of Guardians and Masters of Workhouses at the beginning. Louisa Twining was shocked by the conditions found in the Unions (workhouses), and particularly by the way in which all classes of inmates continued, in spite of the ideas of Chadwick (Finer 1952), to be allowed to mingle together:

'As the work advanced, the various needs of the different classes who formed the heterogeneous populations of workhouses became the subject of thought and discussion as to hopes and endeavours of improvement. The first branch, or division, that seemed to call loudly for help, was that of the able-bodied young girls and women, who, good and bad together, were found to be mixed up in one hopeless class, which was (in the larger London workhouses especially) the despair, and almost terror, of the officials ... Thus arose the desire to obtain the means of rescuing the more hopeful of the young women and girls by taking them away from the workhouse, and, with the sanction of the guardians, placing them in a home apart from these evil associations.'

(Twining 1880:26)

A particular concern for the plight of women in the workhouses led Louisa Twining to the view that women ought to be more closely and integrally involved in the running of workhouses. She felt that women would notice and be sensitive to much 'which no man ought to be expected to discover or control'. In 1860 she gave evidence concerning pauper schools to a Commission on Education, and again stressed the importance of womanly influence:

'I am convinced that *women* should have a greater share in it. No Boards of Guardians, and no officials, can be expected to manage girls' schools as they ought to be, neither can male inspectors alone inspect them. Results would be far different if the influence of women of feeling and education were largely introduced ... and constant lady visitors, who could cultivate the affections of the children and help to counteract the fatal effects of life in an institution and in a mass for girls.' (Twining 1880:33)

Her work was crowned with success when in 1867 a Bill for the reform of workhouses came before Parliament, incorporating provisions for the classification and separation of the heterogeneous population. It took longer for women to gain a foothold in the workhouses in an official capacity:

'Educated women as Guardians, as matrons, as nurses, as inspectors, had been over and over again urged as the one hope of reform and amelioration, ever since the theme was first taken up by Mrs Jameson in her "Lectures on the Social Employments of Women" and "Commission of Labour" in 1855–56. But the idea like many others, had with regard to this point, taken more than the allotted "ten years" to ripen; yet great was the rejoicing when it was found that it was proposed, by the central and all important office to appoint a *lady* as official inspector of all the Metropolitan workhouse and district schools, with the view of gaining evidence upon the conflicting testimony with regard to the system of boarding out orphan pauper children. No more fortunate or judicious appointment could have been made for this first experiment in an untried field than that of the late lamented Mrs Nassau Senior.[2]   (Twining 1880:65)

Concern for pauper children was closely connected with concern for pauper girls and women; both were seen as a natural sphere of interest for middle-class women reformers and philanthropists such as Louisa Twining and Mrs Nassau Senior (daughter-in-law of the economist attacked by Marx). Already, some years earlier Mary Carpenter had begun her work with the children of the very poor in Bristol. She had started a Ragged School in 1839 and this had led her naturally into a wider interest in juvenile delinquents. She wrote her first book on reformatory schools in 1851, called a conference of workers in the field, and this in turn formed a committee to put forward the arguments in favour of having special schools of this kind. The next year the first plans for Kingswood Reformatory School were made, and Mary Carpenter devoted the rest of her life to running this and its companion girls' school, Red Lodge, which was opened not long after.

Mary Carpenter wrote exclusively about the problem of juvenile delinquency, and in her work is found the theme that runs through all such writings at this time; the importance of Home and the Family. In the early Victorian period just as man, wife, and children were often flung apart and the home splintered by the new factory system, so the *Poor Law* in its workings showed that when family conflicted with economic necessity it was ruthlessly split up. In the workhouses there was rigid segregation by sex, while children were parted from their parents. Yet later it was as if these effects of industrialization had themselves awakened the Victorians to a more conscious sense of the functions and importance of the family. And the Family was especially the sphere of women. So Mary Carpenter expressed a widely held view when she wrote that the education and training of pauper girls ought to be:

> '... to make especial efforts to introduce them as completely as possible to what in a well-ordered family would be common domestic duties, to awaken in them healthy affections, and to call out their intellectual powers ... if the girls can be detained under good management, they much more quickly than the boys exhibit a change of demeanour.'
>
> (Carpenter 1853 : 85)

Florence Hill, Octavia's sister, also worked with and wrote about pauper children, 'the children of the State' as she called them, and the same preoccupations are to be found in her writings on the subject:

> 'Among all the endless paradoxes of female treatment, one of the worst and most absurd is that which while eternally proclaiming "home" to be the only sphere of a woman, systematically educates all the female children of the State without attempting to give them even an idea of what a home might be.'   (Hill 1868 : 26)

She described the many schemes being undertaken during the middle years of the century of alternative forms of care for children. Some were apprenticed to manufacturers, with varying results; voluntary homes were set up in many parts of the country, but these were not always successful. A number of Unions set up homes, and later the cottage home came to be regarded as a preferable alternative to the vast, barrack-like institutions. Increasingly also, the solution of boarding out pauper children with respectable working-class foster families seemed to be the very best alternative provided, of course, it was accompanied by active and adequate provision. As Mary Carpenter wrote:

> 'A real good home is infinitely better than any school for the education of girls; even a second rate or a third rate one is preferable. There her true nature is developed and unless she is thus prepared to fill its duties well in after life all other teaching is comparatively useless.'   (Carpenter 1868 : 240)

Since even to become a social worker in those days involved some pioneering spirit, many of the women social reformers were sympathetic to feminism and even involved in the suffrage movement. Whereas the feminist movement of today, as we shall see, challenges many of the assumptions of modern social work, nineteenth century feminism was rather different. It was a call for the rights of women analogous to the claim for the rights of man. It expressed the liberalism of the age, and John Stuart Mill (1869), for example, based his arguments for women's suffrage on those used by the men of the bourgeoisie to obtain their rights and he saw that the subjection of women was out of line with the rest of bourgeois society. Also, the demand for the vote (not yet accorded to the working-class man) and for property rights for women represented a concern for the rights of the women of the bourgeoisie, as Lydia Becker frankly revealed when she wrote:

' "What I most desire is to see men and women of the *middle-classes* stand on the same terms of equality as prevail in the working classes – and the highest aristocracy. A *great lady* or a factory woman are independent persons – personages – the women of the middle classes, are *nobodies*, and if they act for themselves they lose caste!" ' (Rosen 1974:8)

Many of the campaigns of the suffrage movement centred round the needs of these women – for the vote (Rosen 1974), for adequate education (Kamm 1958), for work. Others, such as the efforts to improve the lot of battered women, and, perhaps most important of all, Josephine Butler's campaign for the repeal of the *Contagious Diseases Acts* during the 1860s, touched on the plight of working-class women, whose ills, however, because of the great gulf set between rich and poor, could easily seem quite different from those of the woman of leisure.

The campaign around the *Contagious Diseases Acts* (*1864–1869*) was important because it went beyond philanthropy and bourgeois women's rights. The Acts required the registration and police supervision of women in garrison towns suspected of being prostitutes, and at one time there were many prominent figures both in and outside Parliament who wanted them to extend to cover the whole country. The word of the police was enough for a woman to be registered, and the campaign was fought on the issue not of moral purity but of the deprivation of constitutional rights, although many women who supported the campaign felt that it was in fact unjust for women to be persecuted and victimized on account of 'vice' for which men were held to be primarily responsible. Failing at the outset to get support from prominent friends and the rich, Josephine Butler sought and won support instead from working-class men, Mechanics Institutes, and the like. The significance of this was that it meant that these men saw the issue as a class issue, and as an attempt to foist the slur of prostitute on all working-class women.

The campaign also brought into the open many sexual matters hitherto never spoken of. Social work and nursing too blew away some of the ignorance of Victorian middle-class women, as Henrietta Barnett described:

> 'With the ignorance and enthusiasm of twenty four years [I was] dominated by the faith that no girls liked being wicked, that they had only adopted evil ways inadvertently or under compulsion, and that they would gladly suffer hardship and enjoy discipline so as to become good. Slowly I learnt the truth ... I had arrived at woman's estate in a condition of almost incredible ignorance ... To learn the facts of sex-lawlessness through the channel of the rude words and impure minds of the women in the ... wards of the Whitechapel infirmary made me ill, but I was absorbingly interested in the individual girls ...'   (Barnett 1918:209)

Josephine Butler, in particular amongst the early feminists, had a rich and complex perception of the problems of being a woman. She understood the connection between the unmentionable plight of the fallen woman and the problem of the woman who needed work, for she had seen and known girls in the Liverpool workhouse who had been driven to one by lack of the other. She, like Elizabeth Garrett Anderson, the pioneer woman doctor, was a happily married woman with children, and it was Elizabeth Garrett who wrote that 'the woman question will never be solved in any complete way so long as marriage is thought to be incompatible with freedom and an independent career' (Manton 1965:279). But many of the early feminists did not marry, and their lives offer an often moving and painful example of the triumph of will over emotion; passionate, they repressed their ardour with the scourge of a self-punishing religious devotion, reproaching themselves, as did Mary Carpenter, when, lonely and starved of affection, she sank into the 'selfishness' of depression; managing by strength of character to overcome enormous obstacles in order to achieve great changes in society, yet stifling personal passion on the way, and permitted by society to become more than women at the cost of giving up the womanly claim to personal fulfilment and happiness – at the cost, in other words, of renouncing both sexuality and motherhood.

Yet partly for this very reason they never fully questioned the assumptions about male and female psychology and about the division of labour between men and women as 'natural' made by John Stuart Mill, who in this simply followed the prevailing beliefs of society. Only today, when women are officially allowed to attempt the combination of marriage, career, and motherhood, have the more fundamental problems forced themselves to our attention.

FOUR

Women & the family since
the Second World War

In the previous chapter I suggested that there is a fundamental difference between the feminism of the nineteenth century and the feminism of today, and that a changed analysis of the State and of State welfare provision is a centrally important part of this difference. I have also suggested earlier that only an analysis of the Welfare State that bases itself on a correct understanding of the position of women in modern society can reveal the full meaning of modern welfarism.

Such an analysis has only become possible since the rise of the new feminism, the Women's Liberation Movement, during the last few years. And this new feminism could arise only in a new situation. Part of that situation was the Beveridgean Welfare State. The post-war settlement, of which Beveridge was a part, was in its turn the outcome of the way in which British society was developing during the first half of this century. Before describing this development (particularly as it affected women), however, I propose to discuss the ideological attitudes towards women and the family that were predominant between 1945 and the beginnings of Women's Liberation in the late sixties. This is partly because I wish to counterpose the way in which women have been perceived in recent times to the way in which they were perceived in the Victorian period, and partly because post-war attitudes to women still deeply colour all our assumptions and all the provisions of the modern Welfare State are shot through with them.

A heavy emphasis on the rebuilding of family life after the Second World War implied a return to traditional roles for women. It is not hard to understand why this should have been so, and I shall atempt to explain it in a later chapter. Why, though, did women themselves after enjoying their freedom during the War, return so readily to 'the immaturity that is femininity' (Friedan 1963)? In part the cold war atmosphere of the fifties may account for the quiescence of feminism, at a time when women's rights were likely to be associated with masculinized Soviet women and an alien way of life. The pervasiveness of cold war paranoia in international relations also actually facilitated the ideology of consensus prevalent inside the different sovereign states of the West.

The assumptions of consensus were : that society was evolving towards an ever greater equality in which there was a perpetual process of levelling up through progressive taxation and public welfare spending; that class war was therefore a thing of the past; and that Britain now 'had' the Welfare State. So, for instance, Andrew Shonfield could casually write in the middle of an onslaught on the trades unions : 'Today there is little scope for improvement in workers' living standards through a further process of redistribution' (1958 : 19).

But the element of consensus I wish to emphasize – because it has consistently been missed out – was the belief that the sex war, like class warfare, was also dead. Just as workers now had the Welfare State and huge wages, so women 'had' the vote – they 'had' equality. As late as 1964 J. A. and Olive Banks could confidently write of feminism as 'a spent force' (1964). Indeed, what was continually emphasized was that, having won emancipation, women were rejecting it, and continued to put marriage and child-rearing first:

'In 1956 the *Economist* published an article entitled "the feminists mop up" in which it was said, "More than a century after Florence Nightingale staged her passionate revolt against the trivial domestic round here are the mass of women still preoccupied with their love-life, clothes, children and homes – all the stuff of the women's magazines ... The ordinary woman persists in the belief that in marriage one ounce of perfume is still worth a peck of legal rights and her dreams of power still feature the femme fatale rather than the administrative grade of the Civil Service. The working class woman especially is almost untouched by the women's movements." '

(Gavron 1968 : 46)

At the same time it was suggested that women now had a choice and freedom never before experienced, and stress was laid on her new, or at least more consciously emphasized, role as consumer:

'Liberated at an early age from cradle-watching, spending not only the household's money but "her own" (one third of wives, twice the 1939 proportion having jobs), fashion's eager slave, the woman of the Fifties possessed at once the time, the resources and the inclination to bring to perfection the new arts of continuous consumption. She was the essential pivot of the People's Capitalism and its natural heroine.'

(Hopkins 1963 : 324)

This crude journalistic expression of a common view, written with the coy facetiousness which often overcomes male commentators when they write about women, points quite accurately all the same to women's important role after the war as consumer, or spender of the man's wage packet. Increased consumer spending was encouraged as part of Keynesian economic policies (to generate demand), and moreover a tendency for the accumulation of material possessions could be seen as one solution, though a false one, to the social and psychological problems of life in capitalist society (Hobsbawm 1968a).

The emphasis on the over-riding importance of women's role in the home as wife and mother, and the emotional value given this role, masked the backward and therefore peculiar nature of housework and its economic value to the employer as a cheap way of servicing the worker. It also masked women's usefulness as a reserve of cheap and docile labour. It was said that women only worked for pin money; this meant that any job the wife and mother might do would be fitted in with her household duties. There seemed little general understanding of the strain this imposed on women who effectively worked an eighty or ninety hour week. A study carried out by the Christian Economic and Social Research Foundation (1957) was one of the few even to suggest a different interpretation. This small survey stressed the bleak poverty that drove young mothers and wives out to work. It also pointed out that poor housing caused many of the difficulties experienced by the women interviewed, and found that a move away from cramped accommodation to a council estate, although welcomed, could mean renewed and greater anxieties, and caused considerable strain in the large number of cases where the higher rent could only be paid by skimping on food and other necessities. Of the 59 mothers at work only three spent *any* of their earnings on their own clothes or make-up, and in most cases the women worked in order to buy basic necessities. Cars were never mentioned, and where the wife's earnings did go towards something above the barest minimum it was towards 'extras' such as a holiday, better food, or much needed furniture. In only very few cases was the wife's boredom at home mentioned and in no cases did the wife mention any liking for her (usually unskilled) work, although she might turn out to enjoy the companionship. It was perhaps not surprising if these women found their work unexciting, for most of them had been trained to a higher level of skill than the jobs they were now doing. This is significant, for it points to the usefulness of married women in the working force – who else will do the worst, unskilled, most badly paid jobs for the community but immigrants and women (and often it is immigrant women). And when we ask why women are prepared thus to lower their expectations the answer is immediately obvious in the higher value they are expected to place on their family role. Just as men, whether they are actually working or not, are defined by their place as workers, (a fact reflected in social security provision – the four week rule, attempts to get lone fathers to place their children in care and go back to work (George and Wilding 1972b) and so on), so women are defined, whether they work or not, by their role in the family and are essentially seen as being at home.

The lives of working wives and mothers were lives in which work was actually unending. One French study (Chombart de Lauwe 1963) showed that working housewives performed a total of about eighty-four hours work a week, while even non-working housewives did a total of between fifty-four and seventy-eight hours; the amount of work rising abruptly with the advent of the first child – in fact only childless wives did as 'little' work as fifty-four hours. One of the few studies to admit that a problem existed (Myrdal and Klein 1956) assumed without question that women would continue to struggle along with their 'two roles' of wage earner and house-wife/mother, and could offer no constructive suggestions other than that management should make working conditions as flexible as possible for married women workers. They thought it must be accepted that women would have to take *fifteen or twenty years* off for child rearing, and that this would have to be 'taken into account' when they went back to work. This was a useless suggestion for professional women, around whom much of the discussion centred at the time. And this 'new' problem of the educated housewife masked the perennial problem of the female wage slave at the bottom of the economic ladder. And what, effectively, could management do to help her, in a society in which it was (and is) assumed that women must care for children with fathers playing at best a very secondary role. One widely praised scheme to help mothers back to work, set up by the Peek Frean biscuit factory in Bermondsey (Jephcott 1962) appeared, significantly, to rely for its success to a great extent on the continued existence of an earlier form of close knit extended family in a small, cohesive community.

The discovery that such communities still existed amongst the working class was a feature of the sociology of the period, which in general, while blind to the problems of women, concentrated on the minutiae of family relationships (Townsend 1957; Young and Willmott 1958; Bott 1957). The family was described as the repository of affectionate feelings, of emotionality, the locus of all human love and feeling, and also as retaining the task of child socialization in the formative years. An overview of the literature summed up the class differences in marriage styles:

'Given a continuous range of behaviour between the extremes of "segregation" and "partnership" (in marriage relationships) it seems clear that there is a strong tendency in modern contemporary marriage to the latter extreme. We recall that it is this change that Young and Wilmott describe as "one of the great transformations of our time, reflecting the improvements in standards of living and the rising status of women".' (Rosser and Harris 1965:205)

This belief, that a 'middle-class' pattern of the marriage relationship as an equal partnership was prevailing, meshed in with the belief that class differences were more or less a thing of the past, and with the belief too that women had achieved equality within the context of an exclusive and even symbiotic marriage relationship. This, they suggested, to a large extent replaced for the woman her female relations (mothers and sisters especially) and for the man his workmates, the togetherness of the bourgeois marriage vitiating these two sources of working-class strength.

Psychologists took a more polemical stance – although this too was supposedly based on scientific enquiry – and urged women to return to or to remain in the home. The theme of latch-key children was taken up in the popular press and neglectful working mothers, their values perverted by materialism and greed for more and more possessions, were blamed for juvenile delinquency. John Bowlby (1963) was the name most closely associated with these views, although his work was simply a slightly popularized expression of the theories that had come from the psychoanalytic influence on fashions in child-rearing beginning to be influential before the war, and which had been reinforced by Britain's war experience of evacuation. His work drew criticism from Barbara Wootton (1959) and more recently has been theoretically attacked (Rutter 1971, 1976). Comer 1974) from several different quarters. Yet, although Bowlby's original research has been shown to be shaky, to say the least, this has not inhibited its continued influence, particularly on social work.

Critics of Bowlby have never denied that babies – and children and adults – need warm, continuing relationships and that affection is essential in the context both of long term sexual and of child-rearing relationships. What has caused disagreement is his picture of a stifling and possessive love, and the narrowly defined role of woman as mother. The kind of family life described in some of the literature (Bell and Vogel 1961) seems claustrophobic, and indeed this literature which focuses almost exclusively on the difficulties of life in the nuclear family suggests implicitly that the enclosed nuclear family intensifies the child's dependency on a very few individuals unnecessarily and thus makes it exceptionally vulnerable. Bowlby, like other psychoanalysts, has implied that in motherhood – and in no other role or relationship – pleasure principle and reality principle coincide, and that the mother's *duty* of reproduction is simultaneously her highest pleasure and source of fulfilment. Freud (1950; 1974; see Horney (1973) for an alternative psychoanalytic view) himself, indeed, said that the woman's penis envy could not be fully compensated until she had a male baby in her arms, since the male child symbolized the penis she envied but had never had. Thus he implicitly placed a higher and more permanent value on the mother–son relationship than on the heterosexual marriage relationship, seen as fraught with ambivalence, while the relationship of mother and daughter was still more coloured by hostility and suppressed homosexuality.

Biological determinism lurks behind these kinds of arguments and the equation of motherhood with pleasure (a different statement from simply recognizing that most women enjoy being mothers at least some of the time) has been particularly confusing in our society at a time when emphasis has been increasingly laid on the duty of sexuality, the duty of pleasure. The promised bliss of the orgasm sugar-coats the pill of the nuclear family. Among the reasons why young women marry at an earlier age is that marriage promises, or an engagement permits, sexual fulfilment – or so at least they hope.

Throughout the fifties public attitudes towards sexual behaviour remained puritanical while managing to incorporate this new emphasis. Women's role in servicing the worker was extended to the duty of welcoming and responding to his love-making. Whereas Eliot Slater and Moya Woodside (1951) in the forties had discovered that large numbers of working-class couples would have thought it 'unseemly to be lustful' and many men and even more women had low – or no – expectations so far as their sexual life was concerned, by the fifties sexual potency in men and sexual responsiveness in women began to be seen as explicitly desirable qualities, emphasized for instance in such opinion moulders as the problem pages of women's magazines. Yet while making greater relaxation, freedom, and pleasure possible for some couples, it could equally add to the ambivalences and tensions of family life, since the higher the degree of sexual ecstasy expected within a domestic relationship, the less fulfilling the life-long monogamous union appeared. The search for sexual fulfilment might indeed, it was feared, lead to promiscuity and higher divorce rates. Mary MaCarthy (1960) went so far as to suggest that in the United States, at least, sexual fulfilment was beginning to be seen as a preferable *alternative* to work for women. She quoted research studies being carried out which suggested that college educated women were less likely to 'achieve orgasm' than their working-class sisters (although Kinsey's findings contradict this); and frigidity in the Freud-soaked atmosphere of the time was serious indeed, for heterosexual fulfilment was *the* touchstone of 'maturity' and femininity. One more task was added to the woman's burden, and now the career woman as well as the wife and mother had to prove herself not only as gifted or at least efficient, but as attractive, sexually desirable, and 'normal' as well. Although it is hard to see it in this way, this was an intensification of female exploitation. That it *is* difficult for women to understand their own aspirations towards desirable femininity as a form of exploitation is because gender-linked behaviour is instilled at a very early age, almost from birth, and is an ingrained and deep-rooted part of our consciousness. To state this is not to launch a puritanical attack on sexual pleasure, but simply to point to its ambivalence within a relationship of oppression and in a male-defined society.

Two Royal Commissions, that on Divorce in 1951, and the Wolfenden Committee in 1957, showed that in Britain the State was preoccupied with even this most private aspect of life. The Morton Commission on divorce was straightforwardly reactionary in its findings (see McGregor (1957) for an informed and witty commentary). Of more interest was the *Wolfenden Report* (1957), which, hailed as progressive when it appeared, actually elaborated upon a newer and more sophisticated repressive ideology. The fifties were haunted by fears of homosexuality. In this country the decade opened with what then seemed the appalling scandal of the Lord Montagu/Pitt Rivers affair. Three men from the upper reaches of society served prison sentences after their alleged lovers from 'an altogether different walk of life' had been induced to turn King's evidence (Wildeblood 1958). The class-ridden aspect of the drama now seems typical of this period of British social history. Both here and in the United States, moreover, homosexuality came to be connected with spying and treason and was one of the cardinal sins of the McCarthy era. Although perceived as liberal and even daring, the Wolfenden recommendations conformed to the ideology of Bowlby and the whole social work and psychiatric approach in seeking to remove homosexuality from the realm of crime and sin only in order to place it instead in the category of mental illness, where it has stayed ever since. It was given no validity or authenticity; and this Report, like all other post-war government reports relating to social policy in any form, seemed primarily concerned with the quality of family life. It rather reluctantly reached its conclusion that male homosexual acts (other than with minors) should be removed from the category of crime only after satisfying itself that this would not lead to the break up of the family, which was regarded as the 'basic unit of society'. And it hastened to reassure the public that its recommendation 'should not be taken as saying that society should condone or approve male homosexual behaviour'. This recommendation had to wait ten years before coming law. But the Committee's repressive recommendations on prostitution were rapidly implemented. It was thought essential to get prostitutes off the streets, and the Committee's recommendations in practice facilitated the organization of call-girl services and the rationalization and greater organization of prostitution – by men, naturally – so that these women had even less control over their lives than before.

In the sixties came other, contradictory influences to change the social fabric. The best positive definition of the Permissive Society is found in the *Finer Report* (1974) which, although it expresses a view many women might find over-optimistic, to say the least, nevertheless expresses that view well. The view of women is a reformist, liberal humanist one typical of the atmosphere of the mid-sixties rather than of the seventies, yet paradoxically in the sixties it would not have been possible to write of women in quite this way:

'The 1950s and 1960s witnessed the cumulative removal of customary and legal restraints upon certain forms of sexual behaviour and upon their public portrayal in print or by the visual arts or for commercial purposes. Legal restrictions on the freedom of married people to escape from the bonds which used to be defended as essential safeguards for the integrity of monogamous marriage have been relaxed, and the sexual freedom of men and women has been enlarged. Some think of these developments as creating a "permissive society"; for others they represent no more than tardy social and legislative adaptation to new knowledge and to new notions of desirable relations between men and women within and without marriage. From whatever angle these changes may be viewed, they cannot be interpreted merely in terms of the more freely visible and often grotesque commercial exploitation of sex which is now making available cheaply to the whole male population the gratifications purchased dearly by the well-off in earlier generations. One result has been to confer new powers of self-direction upon women, so that the double standard of sexual morality retains little vitality in law or in life. When Victorian parents told their daughters about to be married that they were making their beds and would have to lie on them they spoke the precise truth. Wives were then held in marriage by legal, economic and theological bonds; the bonds of matrimony were bonds indeed. These have now dissolved into ties of choice, and modern marriages are sustained by affection or by loyalty or by use and wont. The discipline of marriage has become the consent of the partners and derives no longer from external compulsions. The family has evolved into a democratic institution ...'   (*Finer Report* Vol I 1974:7)

Why was it under a Labour Government that the Permissive Society flowered? Robin Blackburn (1971) has suggested that it was partly because liberal reforms such as divorce, abortion, and homosexual law reform could be offered as sops to Labour's middle-class constituency. They cost nothing, and screened Labour's failure to bring about any kind of economic improvement. A relaxation in sexual morality distracted attention from pressing social and economic problems.

For the first time in the sixties, too, a new form of fertility control, the Pill, discovered accidentally, made it easier for women to fulfil themselves sexually, although their sexuality was still defined in male terms. The partial relaxation in the laws relating to abortion represented by the 1967 Act, and the NHS (*Family Planning*) Act, also passed in 1967, implied something more complex than liberal concessions in any case. Under the new family planning legislation contraceptives were to be widely available and were to be free for the poorest families (just one of many selective benefits introduced during this period). This was an attempt at a population policy and coincided with renewed attacks on large 'problem' families. A view of the Pill as a method of *controlling* young women has indeed gained ground since then, and this can be seen most clearly in the *Finer Report*, where an insistence on a repressive form of fertility control stands out the more clearly by contrast with the surrounding liberalism:

'We urge that the concept of "the best years for child-bearing" be examined by those responsible for family planning services with reference to the desirability on medical, psychological, social and economic grounds of incorporating specific advice about the timing of pregnancy into courses in health and social education directed to the young ...

Professor T. C. N. Gibbens, of the Institute of Psychiatry, London University, drew upon his long experience of the attitudes and behaviour of promiscuous maladjusted girls and the social effects of unwanted pregnancies ... The main arguments for the use of contraception in such cases were that the children of single maladjusted girls were frequently disadvantaged and themselves maladjusted, and that attempts to reduce promiscuity by confinement and control led to greater hysteria, agitation and maladjustment; a more stable life could perhaps be atttained if girls had some degree of freedom to establish relationships, protected from pregnancy ... [The DHSS Survey on Family Planning services, 1973] distinguishes three groups of women more prone than others to have unwanted pregnancies; they are women who marry under the age of 20; those who conceived prenuptially; and the wives of the least skilled workers. We have shown ... the extent to which the first two of these three categories of mothers both overlap and experience significantly higher rates of marriage breakdown than those affecting the generality of married women. Of course the likelihood that such women will be married to unskilled workers is also high ... Special measures will be required to reach some of these groups; domiciliary services in particular may be useful for these reluctant to attend clinics or to consult their general practitioners ... We recommend that those responsible for designing ... family planning policies should give special attention to the groups in the population statistically most likely to produce illegitimate children and high rates of marriage breakdown.'   (*Finer Report* Vol I 1974:486–88)

This passage may seem admirably rational on a first reading. That indeed is part of the trouble, that it is an attempt to foist supposedly rationalistic planning and foresight on a group of women who for the most part have been educated to think of themselves as reaching maturity when they marry and give birth, and for whom motherhood may represent the most fulfilling part of a life pinched by poverty and where the only alternative would be unskilled and badly paid work. Women who fail to limit their families or who conceive in adolescence, before marriage, are not necessarily maladjusted. Theirs may represent the best adaptation possible to the very limiting circumstances of their life. The passage also embodies unthinking assumptions about female sexuality that many have begun to question. A boy or young man would never be described as maladjusted simply because he was 'promiscuous' – whatever that is. Moreover an insistence by social planners and psychiatrists on use of the Pill has often gone with an indifference to its possibly dangerous consequences.

In some ways the most noticeable manifestations of the Permissive Society – the clothes, the music, the property speculation – represented a commercial free-for-all, an expansion of capitalistic frenzy into new spheres ripe for exploitation. New, semi-creative trades catered for new markets – the young, women, increasingly well-off white collar workers, the unmarried young, the teenagers, who collectively had the spending of vast sums of money. There have been endless debates over the value, or otherwise, of youth culture, both in its earlier phase and as it developed and merged into the alternative culture and the Underground. But, revolutionary attack or parasitic alternative, the cultural developments of the sixties offered no new real freedom for women. Jeff Nuttall, for instance, whose book *Bomb Culture* (1970) is the most complete and thought-out expression of the more extreme elements in the alternative culture displays a naively reactionary attitude towards women (remarks such as 'everybody but the wives went upstairs to talk' are typical). The work of Ronnie Laing, which both came from and fed into this culture, was equally blind to the problems of women (see especially Laing and Esterson 1971). Laing's work with and writings on schizophrenics and their families was hailed as revolutionary, yet in his paradigm of the sick family it is usually the mother who turns out to be, effectively, the originator of the madness. The devouring, hostile mother, giving her children double messages and thus confusing them psychologically, over-protecting them, living out her own incipient madness in them by driving them insane is a new form of the medieval conception of the devouring feminine principle – the witch. The men in Laing's families usually seem less sinister, more often inadequate than actively malignant. But if Laing's descriptions appear anti-feminist in blaming women as mothers for their destructive effect on their children, this reflects what actually happens to many women in today's society; that, no alternative role being offered them, they will inevitably try to live through their children. It is not so much that Laing's work was actively or intentionally anti-women as that his books entirely lacked a pointed and explicit analysis of the place of women in our society.

The songs of the Beatles and the Rolling Stones suggested a more conscious and aggressive domination over women. The

Underground had nothing to offer women except a new form of repression. There was no move away from the definition of women as sexual objects rather than sexual beings. Drop-out men may have tried to develop for themselves more 'feminine' attitudes of passivity, receptivity, gentleness, but, to give up traditional male role playing in all other respects seemed often to leave them with a need for reassurance in sexual relationships that they were still men. In the magazines of the Underground, in *Oz*, *Frendz*, and *IT*, sexism simply reached a new level of hysteria.

FIVE

Welfare since the War

Attitudes to women, like class attitudes, as part of the ideology of our society, were bound to be reflected in post-war welfare provision, given that social policy always contains an ideological component. Forming a link between ideology and the economy social welfare has also of course reflected the steadily worsening economic situation since the war (Gough 1975).

The Welfare State as negotiated after the Second World War meant that henceforth the provision by the State of various kinds of social services was to be regarded as part of wages, or at least as an integral part of the wage contract and – along with longer holidays, safety regulations, pensions, and health schemes – as a new bargaining counter in the process of wage struggle. Hence the notion of the 'social wage'. In the early post-war years this was not discussed directly, but in the recent period of crisis the Labour Government has fallen back on this concept and attempted to justify incomes policies and its various attempts to hold down wages by openly including the 'social wage' as part of the whole wage. As Joe Rogaly explained to *Financial Times* readers:

'What Mrs Castle wants is a simple exposition of the nature of the "social wage" put out in a form that everyone can understand. In her view discussions of personal income should not be exclusively in terms of take-home pay. Public services – schools, hospitals, medical attention, social security payments, subsidised housing and transport – should also be expressed as a form of income. In times of rapid inflation excessive cash wage demands can of course jeopardise the "social wage" – and I suppose that the assumption is that if everyone knew this and understood it they might behave differently.'   (8.7.1975)

Denis Healey in his 1975 Budget speech calculated the social wage at £1,000 per head per annum, yet a recent Counter Information Services Special Report on the Cuts (1975) has broken down the £1,000 and demonstrated that much of it goes on arms spending and other forms of non-welfare spending. It is perhaps easier to emphasize the 'social wage' in the hope of restraining wage demands than to attempt to cut State welfare expenditure which has had an inborn tendency to grow in recent times. For one thing population trends have meant that there are proportionately more dependent members of the population and fewer working members. (The share of social services going to the old has risen in all West European countries since the War.) The relationship between the birthrate and the economic structure is not fully understood but certainly the low birthrate between the Wars was due in part to the conditions of the depression and has resulted in the proportionately small working force since 1945. A low birthrate also leads to demands for higher standards of maternity and educational service for the children that are being born. Another reason for rises in social expenditure is the nature of modern capitalism and what R. M. Titmuss (1968) has called the 'diswelfares' produced by modern urban industrial societies, with much welfare provision representing partial compensation for the social costs – for instance increased chronic sickness amongst older workers (*see* Abel Smith and Townsend 1965; Kinkaid 1973) – of capitalism rather than outright benefits. Amongst these are diswelfares in terms of the social cost to the family. Night work and the 'twilight shift' eat away at the fabric of family life, and even day work on a speeded up assembly line can have similar effects:

> ' "I never thought I'd survive. I used to come home from work and fall straight asleep. My legs and arms used to be burning. And I knew hard work. I'd been on the buildings but this place was a bastard then. I didn't have any relations with my wife for months. Now that's not right, is it? No work should be that hard." '
>
> (Benyon 1973 : 75)

Economic need and the position of women have reinforced each other more directly in some areas of welfare provision than in others. Often, as I have already suggested, the position of women was an ignored but vital part of social problems. For instance the whole way in which poverty was discussed in the post war period neglected the particular ways in which poverty – low income – particularly effects women.

Poverty itself was however exhaustively discussed. In the fifties, in the context of the 'Affluent Society' (Galbraith (1958) is one of the most influential exponents of this theory) it was widely believed that poverty had disappeared. This myth was welcomed by both Tories and Labour, the Tories because it meant that Tory freedom worked, the Labour Party because it meant that the Welfare State worked. The disappearance of poverty was 'proved' by Seebohm Rowntree (1951) who in 1950 undertook a third survey of York (to follow up his earlier studies of 1899 (published 1901 and 1941 respectively) and 1936), and, placing his poverty line at thirty six per cent higher than the level of National Assistance benefits, found that the proportion of the total population living in poverty was now 1.5 per cent compared with 18 per cent in 1936. He also found that those still in poverty were mainly the old, and large families. He attributed this striking change to Beveridge, that is to full employment and the Welfare State. What it actually showed, however, was that there was full employment, for

Beveridge had been precisely supposed to prevent poverty when earnings were interrupted by sickness or old age, and in large families by way of family allowances. 136 per cent of national assistance benefits represents a very low income and leaves untouched vast inequalities of wealth and property ownership, but the usefulness of measuring poverty in this way – by the position of individuals above or below an absolute poverty line instead of in relative terms – is precisely that it enables poverty to be discussed as a residual problem. When attention is focused on special categories of people 'in need', the old, the chronically sick, or one-parent families, it is possible to ignore the fact that their problems are but extreme manifestations of the general pattern of a society dominated by class inequalities and wide differences of wealth. It is possible to forget that 1 per cent of the population owns (approximately) 50 per cent of all privately owned wealth (Atkinson 1974), and that almost all workers are vulnerable to the hazards of poverty at some time in their lives. Seebohm Rowntree had in fact discovered a cycle of poverty in his earlier surveys, which showed that poverty hit individuals and families at specific stages in the life cycle, especially when children were small and again in old age, and was interspersed with periods of relative non-poverty when there was more than one wage earner in the family. And for women this meant often that it was their 'double shift' – paid work plus work in the home – which made possible the relative affluence of their family, while their capacities as mothers were hampered by poverty when their children were small, and while again in old age they were the ones most likely to be suffering, since the majority of old-age pensioners are women.

It was useful politically, however, to see the 'poor' as though this were some sort of special group akin to the physically handicapped, or a minority group such as the blacks or homosexuals because it then became a welfare or cultural problem and could be successfully divorced from class perspective. It was also useful for them to be grouped further within special categories of need, since then their social differences both from the non-poor and also from other groups of poor people, rather than their common economic plight, could be emphasized. The connection of poverty with large families was especially useful, since these could be scapegoated as a feckless, self-indulgent group, this disapproval sharpened by envy of their presumed sexual over-indulgence. (This explanation also plays on racialism, since immigrant groups are popularly supposed to have larger families than other groups.)

In the fifties it was genuinely believed (Galbraith 1958) – as Rowntree appeared to prove – that economic growth and full employment indefinitely continued would be able, if associated with growing productivity, to wipe out poverty. An important feature of the Welfare State as set up after 1945 had been its 'universalism', that it provided a subsistence minimum income as a security floor to prevent destitution, to which all were entitled, without a means test, and thus without stigma. The education and health systems had been set up on the same basis. (This at least had been the theory, although in practice the existence of a continuing private sector in health, education, and insurance prevented the ideal from ever becoming a reality.) However the belief that poverty was disappearing paved the way for attacks on the principle of universalism, which began in the very early fifties (*Economist* 1951; *The Times* 1952; Powell and Macleod 1952).

From the belief that poverty was disappearing it was also only a short step to the assumption that the few remaining poor must be inadequate and even pathological in some way. This belief was elaborated into the ideology of the 'problem family', popular with social workers throughout the decade. These families had already been identified among the evacuees during the War (Hygiene Committee of the Women's Group on Public Welfare 1942), and in 1947 the Eugenics Society sponsored an enquiry into them. Its report quoted several definitions of what a problem family was, relying for an explanation on hereditary defect:

'It is difficult to define such families but one is tempted to borrow from a description of feeble-mindedness, and call them those families "with social defectiveness of such a degree that they require care, supervision and control for their own well-being and that of others" ... A problem family is one that lives in squalor and is content to do so. It apparently suffers from domestic and possible social ineducability. Its members may be distinguished by lack of character and by mental backwardness, sometimes associated with relatively numerous children, child neglect, intemperance etc.' (C. P. Blacker 1947 : 14)

Philip Seed (1973) has suggested that problem families became a scapegoat of the fifties because they were 'a sore thumb held downwards in front of the cheery face of the Welfare State'. They reminded Britain that the poor *were* still around, and so they had to be explained away as pathological deviants, the last survivors of a state of things that had disappeared rather than as the tip of any iceberg.

Some sociologists (for example, Peter Townsend) always argued that poverty had by no means disappeared, but it was not until the 1960s, when growing inflation and unemployment began slowly to make it impossible to ignore, that the public 'rediscovery of poverty' found expression in a number of studies (HM Government 1967a; Atkinson 1969), in particular *The Poor and the Poorest* by Brian Abel Smith and Peter Townsend published in 1965. The response of social policy to this changed perception of the extent, and even to some degree the' nature of poverty was an increasing move away from universalism and towards selectivity, towards earnings related social security benefits to soften the blow of redundancies due to the modernization of capital (George 1973) and towards an increased emphasis on special categories of people with a claim to social benefits. The 1970 Tory Election Manifesto, for example, enshrined its selectivist approach in a section headed 'Care for those in Need', and the trend henceforth was to be away from a national guaranteed minimum for all and towards benefits primarily for special groups.

From Speenhamland onwards levels of benefits to the unemployed have always borne a relation to the low wage sector, and the persistence of low wages has had the effect that benefits must remain even lower. In particular, women's position as claimants is related to their position as low paid workers and caught between this and their official definition as primarily mothers, they come off very badly when left to the mercy of the State social security system. This has been true throughout the post-war period. In 1958 Peter Marris (1958) described in often grim and tragic terms the plight of women and children when the increasingly fragile fabric of the nuclear family is broken, in this case by widowhood. A forward to Marris's book by John Bowlby stressed the plight of the children; equally horrifying was the plight of the widowed mothers thrown back on state pension or supplementary benefit, a prey to loneliness, social isolation, and sexual deprivation, and expected to fulfil a double role towards their children. Even with the support of the extended family, all the weaknesses of the woman's dependent position was clearly revealed. Nor have matters changed nearly twenty years later. The *Poverty Reports* for both 1974 and 1975 (Young) emphasized that into whatever category they came, women have been the most hard done by amongst the poor and welfare claimants. Michael Young's mini-survey of Bethnal Green carried out in the autumn of 1973, showed that:

'What stands out most sharply is the plight of the women. Even when married, if they were tied to the home by young children and unable to work themselves, there was very far from any guarantee that their "wages" from the husband would keep pace with his. When not married but with children dependent on them, their lot was still less enviable.'

(Young 1974:128)

and a year later their plight had not improved:

'There is not yet any sign of any fundamental change having been made ... Of the ninety-six households in the Camden survey who were in poverty 70 per cent were headed by women. They predominated amongst the old and amongst single parents. In Camden too, one out of every three non-working wives had not had any increase during the year in the housekeeping allowance received from their husbands. This meant that their real income went down, which was specially serious for those with young children to maintain in poor families. This finding serves as yet another reminder that *mothers and children can be in poverty while husbands are not* ... Disabled housewives are treated by the government's new disability scheme as if they did not exist.'

(Young 1975:15)

Moreover these findings have been borne out by larger surveys. As reported in the *Financial Times*:

> 'Many wives are not benefiting from their husbands' pay
> rises ... At least one in five husbands has not given his wife
> a rise, although in many cases he has received one. Over half
> the husbands still earning less than £20 a week have been
> unable to increase the housekeeping money over the last 12
> months.
>
> The findings are from a two-part survey commissioned by
> the National Consumer Council to discover whether hidden
> pockets of family poverty are being caused by husbands'
> failure to pass on a share of higher wages. The survey
> covered 4,000 questionnaires returned by readers of Woman's
> Own and 1,830 interviews carried out by National Opinion
> Polls.
>
> Both samples show that a significant minority of husbands
> have failed to give their wives a housekeeping rise. According
> to the Woman's Own sample, one in five is managing on the
> same budget as last year even though 58 per cent of husbands
> have been given a rise since then. Nationally this would
> mean that more than 2 million wives have 20p less in the
> pound in real terms.
>
> The NOP sample suggests that wives are having an even
> tougher time – with one in four husbands failing to increase
> the housekeeping allowance.
>
> Both samples indicate that the poorer the family the less
> likely is the wife to have had a rise.'   (17.9.1975)

Most notorious of all welfare provisions affecting women remains the cohabitation ruling. Claimants Unions (Highbury and
Islington Claimants Union 1971) and the Child Poverty Action
Group (Lister 1973; Streather and Weir 1974) have attacked it.
Olive Stevenson (1972) writing in her capacity as social work
adviser to the DHSS was also critical of its workings, even
though her point of view reflects the mainstream of social
work thinking in concentrating on the psychological inadequacies of claimants. The argument used by the SBC to justify
the cohabitation ruling was that it would be wrong to treat a
woman living with a man but not married to him differently
from a married woman, and, since a married woman cannot
claim supplementary benefits for herself, her husband must do it

for both of them, therefore the single woman too must be treated as if economically dependent on the man with whom she is living. Any other ruling would be a discouragement to marriage. Olive Stevenson suggests that this analysis is irrefutable 'within the framework of existing social and moral conventions', but does recognize that some would question those conventions. She, however, relates this rather to what she perceives as changing sexual customs (i.e. the Permissive Society) and a greater tolerance towards unmarried couples who live together, rather than to feminist values. She is aware that 'the moral value ... contained in the cohabitation rule [is] ... that a shared household with a woman carried with it for the man a financial responsibility comparable to that of marriage' (1972 : 143). But, while aware of the implication of the cohabitation ruling, she never questions whether *marriage itself* should contain these same elements of breadwinner and dependant.

In fact, the cohabitation ruling only embodies in slightly more glaring form the innermost assumption of marriage which is still that a man should pay for the sexual and housekeeping services of his wife. We are so accustomed to this that it seems natural within marriage; the cohabitation rule and its enforcement simply draw back the veil from the general reality of sexual relations within our society, which are, and must remain, distorted and contaminated so long as marriage – like prostitution – remains an *economic* option for women, a job. So far as cohabitation itself goes, the low tactics to which special investigators (or sex snoopers as even the right-wing press has called them) will sink have been well documented. Yet after the Fisher Committee in 1972 had investigated alleged abuse of social security and found that there was remarkably little of it, the Tory Government's response was to increase the number of special investigators; while the cosmetic operation carried out in March 1976 does nothing to change the ruling, but simply suggests it should be administered more courteously!

If the cohabitation ruling embodies the belief that women should depend on men, State education since the War has tried to bring them up so that they should be equipped to do this and not much else. Education has more generally been a British obsession since World War Two and is closely connected with beliefs about social control and the family as well as the role of women. Educationalists have themselves talked of an obsession, and John Vaizey for example thought the cause of the obsession was the importance of education today as 'virtually *the* avenue for social mobility'. He noted too the new centrality of the 'classless' family:

'Take the growth in the strength of family life, for instance. The serious-minded husband and wife, buying their house on a mortgage, rearing the well-dressed children you see all over the country, are deeply concerned that their children shall get a good start in life. Of course one can sneer at this; "Keeping up with the Joneses", "Death in a suburb" and so on. But compared with life in the Orwellian slums of the thirties or the Wellsian small-shopkeeper existence in Edwardian days, this new way of living (new only in that it is *the* typical way of life) is in almost every way better.'

(Vaizey 1962:10)

There have been a number of important Government Reports on education in the period since the war. The earlier Reports, *Crowther* in 1959 and in 1963 the *Newsom Report*, *Half our Future*, which dealt with the education of pupils between thirteen and sixteen years old, of 'average or less than average' ability, had a definitely ideological attitude towards girls. Both were preoccupied with the social control of youth and saw a solution to this problem in terms of fitting the child to the 'real world' of the kind of work he was likely to perform in adult life. Presumably the assumption behind this idea was that teenage delinquency was caused in part by discontent and that if adolescents lowered their sights and were more consistently initiated into their future station in life as unskilled or at the most semi-skilled workers, then their discontent would be reduced and with it their rebellious behaviour. Visits to factories, the learning of practical skills, and guidance on sexual behaviour were to be part of the school programme in the final year; and for girls this meant training to be a housewife, and an insistence on traditional female roles:

'The Crowther Report ... recommended that "the prospect of courtship and marriage should rightly influence the education of adolescent girls; their direct interest in dress, personal appearance, in problems of human relationships should be given a central place in their education". Later on Katharine Ollerenshaw, a contributor to the Newsom Report wrote "the incentive for girls to equip themselves for marriage and home-making is genetic". Newsom was also important in stating the distinction to be made for the "clever girl". "More able girls," he said, "had no time for education specifically related to their careers as women, but the less able do have".'

(Loftus 1974:8)

For less able, read working class. Sir John Newsom expanded on his beliefs in the *Observer* re-emphasizing, by implication, the development of the intellect as essentially male:

'We try to educate girls into becoming imitation men and as a result we are wasting and frustrating their qualities of womanhood at great expense to the community. I believe that in addition to their needs as individuals, our girls should be educated in terms of their main social function – which is to make for themselves, their children and their husbands a secure and suitable home and to be mothers.'   (6.9.1974)

Yet why, if it is eternally *natural* for girls to be 'home-makers' should an educational system need to *instil* these qualities?

'There may be some girls who are far from enthusiastic, because they have had their fill of scrubbing and washing-up and getting meals for the family at home; and yet, they may need all the more the education a good school course can give in the wider aspects of home-making, and the skills which will reduce the element of domestic drudgery.'

(*Newsom Report* 1963:135)

By the time the *Plowden Report* appeared in 1967 the approach had softened, but only a little. The Plowden Committee saw the solution to the dual role of women as lying in part-time work, and accordingly suggested that nursery provision should be part time too, with full-time nurseries reserved for the 'deprived' child.

Social work even more than education has played, since the War, an expanding and highly ideological role. Its emphasis has been directly on the reinforcement of traditional forms of family life; this has in fact been its main purpose within the constellation of Welfare State services and the reality behind its official role which has tended to be described in terms of the allocation of scarce resources and the personalizing of the impersonal bureaucratic structures which dispense welfare benefits. In the social work literature the family is seen as eternal, unchanging, and ahistorical: 'Family life is perpetuated of itself and by no artificial teaching, and if it is to be kept alive this can only be done by deliberately fostering of its vitality' (Heywood 1959:139). This is an obvious absurdity, but quite typical (it comes from an ordinary, standard textbook on social work in child care), and it well expresses the nervous ambivalence that has been such a feature of public attitudes to the family since the beginnings of the industrial revolution. It is perceived as the essential bedrock of society, yet as threatened and fragile, undermined by the rapidity of change in a technologically advanced society. This essentially nostalgic and pessimistic view may take account of one feature of social change, which is the changing position of women, but can hardly be optimistic or welcoming of it. There is no indication in the social work literature that human beings have any inherent tendencies to form socially cohesive and supportive bonds, or that the new conditions of low birthrate and longer life could, with improved technological conditions, constitute an opportunity for the development of new and more diverse forms of child care and affective relationships. On the contrary there is a constant and lowering atmosphere in which the difficulties of achieving any sort of normal and happy adjustment to life are emphasized. And indeed the task is bound to be difficult since normality and adjustment are defined in rigid and narrow ways.

The theory underlying post-war social work was overwhelmingly that of psychoanalysis. Psychoanalytic casework had first burgeoned in the United States in the 1920s, and in fact it is interesting that while lagging behind in welfare provision generally, America has led the field in the development of a highly ideological theory of social work. It has been suggested (Weinberger 1975) that this development was made possible by the reactionary atmosphere of the United States after the end of the First World War. Then, the Progressive Era (1896–1916) during which many social workers had been active as social reformers, gave way to a period of reaction during which fears of Bolshevism, following the Russian Revolution, and the confidence of big business during a period of boom, combined to produce a situation in which social workers were amongst many other radicals and political activists who faced loss of their jobs (and worse) should they be seen to be allied to the cause of social reform. General prosperity – although countless numbers of individuals remained poor – facilitated the emergence of psychoanalysis as a formative influence on social work. Individuals turned inward to examine their own psyches rather than outward, when this seemed so dangerous. Yet the popularity of Freud requires some explanation in a country like America:

'How could a theory that is pessimistic, non-religious and highly sexual, particularly a theory based on the concept of childhood sexuality, achieve its stronghold in a nation whose intellectual heritage and history eschewed the main thrust of the theory's ideas?' (Weinberger 1975:107)

In other words, how could the determinism of Freud be acceptable in a society that, because of its pioneering history, had always perforce emphasized the conscious power of the individual to better himself and succeed by striving? As a partial solution to this problem, American practitioners inserted into Freud's original theories the Social Darwinist implant of ego-psychology, a more adaptive version of Freud, which places less emphasis on the unconscious and more on the strength and 'realism' of the conscious Ego. (This is in itself a vulgarization, since for Freud himself the conscious Ego was not to be equated with rationality in this uncomplicated way.)

It seems likely that psychoanalysis caught on in the USA because increased prosperity led to increased leisure amongst the upper and middle class at a time when women were becoming 'emancipated'. It may well be that a changing attitude towards women as sexual beings together with the vote, their entry into higher education, but together also with a lack of real equality and job opportunity, led to new conflicts and consequently to an increased preoccupation with women's traditional roles as wife and mother rather than to a real expansion of horizons. This would account for the obsession with scientific approaches to right child rearing:

'The acceptance of psycho-analysis by the upper class, the medical profession, and the intelligentsia (whose members included the college teachers of the educated new women) reinforced women's acceptance of psycho-analytic theory as the scientific elixir for improving the psychic well-being of her family ... Most of the caseworkers of the era were women who could easily identify with the psycho-analytic emphasis espoused by their employing agencies. Since they shared the problems of other emancipated women, many felt that psycho-analysis could help them with their personal problems.'
(Weinberger 1975:107)

That is to say, they accepted the Freudian belief that 'emancipation' was in itself a problem and this had far-reaching and reactionary results. Ultimately it was possible to use Freud's emphasis on psychic development as yet another theory to reinforce the individualism characteristic of the USA, and to identify poverty and other social problems as the fault of individuals.

The 'psychiatric deluge' did not reach its peak of influence in this country until the fifties. In Britain, although it has been an important influence, particularly in psychiatric social work where it was used, amongst other things, to support claims to professional status, it has never achieved the dominance it won in the USA, where perhaps some more unifying theory of personality was needed to forge bridges between different cultures and immigrant groups.

Nevertheless a psychoanalytic approach to personal problems did gain importance after the Second World War when social work assumed a new role. This new role was spelled out in 1948, in the preface to a book brought out by the Family Discussion Bureau. The FDB was an offshoot of what had once been the COS, but had just been renamed the Family Welfare Association. It suggested that now that the Welfare State had dealt with material problems, social workers would be free to promote healthy relationships:

'The setting up of State Welfare services, in particular the implementation of the National Health Act and the National Insurance Acts, had taken over many of the functions hitherto carried out by voluntary welfare agencies, and had freed the Association sufficiently to make the quality of family life and the personal happiness of its clients its primary concern.'   (Pincus 1953:3)

The case histories in the body of the book are filled with amazing success stories, achieved through therapeutic casework, with women 'making astonishing moves towards femininity', and learning to become good mothers, and men rapidly overcoming their effeminacy and homosexual tendencies, achieving new status in work and doubling their earning capacities (see Weir 1975). The authors stress the importance of correct gender identifications and the neurosis and immaturity to which those who fail to become truly 'masculine' or 'feminine' are condemned. Expressing the then current horror of homosexuality, the book expresses open disapproval of effeminate men or, even worse, of women such as Mrs P, 'a very hysterical girl, feminine in appearance but with an immense need to dominate and be masculine' or of Mrs M whose 'successful' treatment is described with naive brutality:

'The progress Mrs M had made was obvious. She had gone a long way towards femininity; she showed a new interest in the home, in sewing and cooking. While ... she seemed pleased about her achievements, she made angry remarks to the (social) worker, suggesting that she wanted to make her into a "humdrum housewife" with washing on Mondays, and a dull, competent routine.'   (Pincus 1953:131)

It is hard not to share Mrs M's suspicions. The whole book, indeed, is like an etiquette manual of the personality – what clothes and manners are appropriate to one's psychological station in life, and how to steer a narrow and perilous course between the rocks of one's unconscious identifications with faulty patterns of parental behaviour on one side and the sirens of acting out and other forms of infantile gratification on the

other. Sexual satisfaction is seen as a goal achieved with difficulty and at the cost of mammoth self denial in other areas of
life.

Another and equally important aspect of social work was its
function in the management of the working-class family in a
more direct way. There was a new emphasis on 'prevention'
which meant that help should be given to families in their own
homes where it was felt that they had difficulty in caring for
their children in a socially acceptable way. Before the War the
social solution to the neglected or delinquent child had been
his removal to an institution, but this was expensive. Home
support was justified in psychological rather than economic
terms, however:

> 'In work with neglectful parents our increasingly organised
> knowledge of the patterns of human behaviour and studies
> of their social and psychological motivation is of vital
> importance. With this knowledge, incomplete and imperfect
> as it is, it begins to be possible for the caseworker to accept
> the historic challenge thrown down by the new approach, to
> change the psychological and social environment of the neg-
> lected child, and by working with the parents, the actual
> makers of the environment, to help them produce that change
> themselves. It thus became possible for the first time to see
> the prevention of neglect as the prevention of deprivation
> too.'   (Heywood 1959:178)

Such views are still widely held amongst social workers today,
and the arrogance of the assumptions underlying such an
approach still go unchallenged all too often.

A Committee to investigate the problems of the delinquent
child was set up in 1956 and from this came the *Ingleby Report*
in 1960. This likewise laid great emphasis on the importance of
supporting and increasing family responsibility and family
strength. Delinquency was defined as a family and not as a social
or economic problem: 'It is often the parents as much as the
child that need to alter their ways, and it is therefore with
family problems that any preventive measures will be largely
concerned' (1960:7). This Report was followed in 1963 by the
Children and Young Persons Act which made it easier for

workers to prevent young children from coming into care, because it was now possible to provide direct cash help, and because the Act meant the official recognition of 'prevention' as a legitimate sphere of work. But since the cash help could only be given if the children were assessed as being liable otherwise to have been received into care, a mother by requesting money laid herself open to constant supervision, inspection, and counselling and to official doubts that she was an adequate mother. Joel Handler (1968) showed that social workers did indeed use these new powers as their chief method of controlling client behaviour and as a way of coercing parents into accepting the social workers' standards of good behaviour. The money was in no way a right, but a highly discretionary benefit and its acceptance did implicitly suggest that the recipient was a bad mother.

The *Younghusband Report* (1959) on the training of social workers also saw the main task of social workers as being to support the family, and explained quite callously how the function of such social work help was to make it possible for individual families to tolerate the absence of social support or adequate health or welfare provision:

'Some individuals or families can carry what is often a very heavy burden of mental or physical sickness or disability in the home over a long period, if they can share some of the stress and strain with someone outside the situation ... In such circumstances the social worker may be required to prevent a general breakdown of family care by giving support and understanding to one or more members, rather than by providing any more concrete form of help.'

(*Younghusband Report* 1959)

In the sixties came a rather different emphasis on the community. The 1959 *Mental Health Act*, for example, envisaged a much wider use of 'community care' for the mentally ill and handicapped, without asking what a community was, or whether modern urban society would continue to throw up close-knit communities of the Bethnal Green type. This Act proposed many forms of support such as day centres, residential hostels, and sheltered workshops; but because these cost money they often failed to materialize, and so in practice community care turned out to mean – the family. And the family in practice turns out to mean primarily the mother, devoting for example, the rest of her life, say forty years, to caring for a mentally handicapped son or daughter, because the institutional alternative is often horrific.

If, in social work, the fifties had seen a conscious attempt to mould family behaviour from early childhood onwards, and to squeeze back into the mould the families who had spilled out of it and become problematical, the sixties, faced with the failure of this approach took the manipulation and management of the working class beyond the family, and whole communities came to be seen as sick and in need of some form of treatment. This form of intervention originated in the United States as part of the attempt to contain the menace of the black ghettoes, but the American War on Poverty defined the problem in terms of bureaucratic breakdown on the one hand and the lethargy and cultural pathology of the client group on the other (Marris and Rein 1970; Titmuss 1968). The British version – social work with families within the context of community development – was enshrined in the *Seebohm Report on Local Authority and Allied Personal Social Services* (1968). This, again, stressed the family as the bulwark against delinquency and took as its jumping off point an earlier White Paper, *The Child, the Family and the Young Offender* (1965), but the *Seebohm Report* went further than the White Paper in that it planned the increased organization of the community as an additional and now much needed reinforcement of the social order:

'Powerful social control may, of course, stifle the individual and produce over conformity, but it has been suggested that the incidence of delinquency is likely to be highest either where little sense of community and hence little social control exists, or where in a situation of strong social control the predominant community values are, in fact, potentially criminal. Such ideas point to the need for the personal social services to engage in the extremely difficult and complex task of encouraging and assisting the development of community identity and mutual aid, particularly in areas characterised by rapid population turnover, high delinquency, child deprivation and mental illness rates and other indices of social pathology. Social work with individuals alone is bound to be of limited effect in an area where the community environment itself is a major impediment of healthy development.'

(Seebohm Report 1968 : 15)

Old communities had been bombed and bulldozed away. They had perhaps seemed threatening to the social order during the Depression when, at times, government had been faced with the organized strength of whole communities, Glasgow, Jarrow, the East End. Now the State faced different problems of social breakdown in the disintegrating communities and new estates alike, so that new forms of social containment were seen as being needed to deal with the unfamiliar and alarming discontents of the children of the Welfare State who had grown up on the new estates and gone to the new schools yet seemed no less destructive and rebellious than their parents. Indeed while less directly politically threatening to the social order than the organizers of the General Strike, the Jarrow marchers or the anti-Fascists, the teenage folk devils (Cohen 1972) seemed at times even more alarming for that very reason, that they did not represent organized politics, but rather the anarchic unreason unleashed by unconscious forces.

Social work was an important form of social containment intended to deal with these new problems. While the *Seebohm Report* did stress the need for more resources and the particular importance of better housing it was written on the assumption that material resources would not in fact be forthcoming : 'An effective family service cannot be provided without additional resources. It would be naive to think that any additional resources will be made available in the near future' (1968 : 15). Social workers, however, were cheaper than new housing or larger social security payments, and social work was one of the few growth industries during the late sixties and early seventies. Their ideological role in particular became both more important and also more exposed in the threatening climate of economic crisis, unemployment, social decay, and generalized unrest. Clearly they *were* being employed partly to reinforce the two concepts that have dominated industrial society and formed the basis of ruling-class ideology : the family and the work ethic. At the same time, the worsening economic situation made their efforts manifestly weak and inadequate and the consequent disillusionment coupled with worsening conditions on the job and the changed political climate, especially among students, has led to a re-politicization of social work so that during the seventies social workers have been in continuous lively debate as to the nature of their work, and, under the barrage of 'theories' on deprivation, cultural poverty, and violence, have themselves regained some of the zeal for social reform found in the Victorian pioneers. A new sophistication has meant that they are less embedded in their own ideology than was the case in the fifties, and this new sophistication reflects a changed relationship to their work. For many social workers the creation of the new, big 'Seebohm factories' (the big amalgamated social services departments set up as a result of the *Seebohm Report*) meant an intensification of their labour. Equipped with a casework training and wholeheartedly liberal ideals (Pearson 1973) they found that the reality of their work was to be a mixture of bureaucratic detail and large-scale economic problems. In response to this there developed in the late sixties a new, 'radical' social work. Some of this radicalism was bourgeois and reformist, seeking for example to emphasize welfare rights rather than emotional problems; or seeking in community work a path away from the manipulation of individuals, although this was one unfortunately that could easily lead to the manipulation of grass-roots groups and protest instead. *Case Con*, inaugurated in 1970, took up a more overtly socialist and revolutionary stance, although it at times seemed to deny that emotional distress existed at all. Both the bourgeois radical and the socialist critiques contained much that was progressive. Both were equally backward in recognizing the special problems of women. As late as 1975 it was still possible for there to appear in a book allegedly about 'radical' social work, an attack on women in the profession on the grounds of their innate conservatism (Jones 1975). Due to their socialization and lack of masculine personality traits they lack, it seems, 'the drive, assertion and commitment necessary for direct action'. Not until 1974 did *Case Con* run a Women's Issue. By this time, as we shall see, the influence of the Women's Movement had begun to make itself felt.

The mainstream of theoretical and ideological work has continued to develop in such a way that traditional views on family life could continually be reintroduced in more sophisticated forms. An example of this would be the 'Cycle of Deprivation', of which the Family Income Supplement was one practical expression. The Cycle was explained by Sir Keith Joseph, when he was the Minister at the DHSS in an interview to the *Guardian* as follows:

> 'Sir Keith's ideas ... begin with the thought that maybe there is a certain "minimum capacity" in parenthood below which children start to suffer ... "Deprivation takes many forms and they interact," he said in a speech to the Pre-Schools Playgroups Association. "It shows itself ... in poverty, in emotional empoverishment, in personality disorder, in poor educational attainment, in depression and despair." The most vulnerable – those at the bottom of the economic and social scales – are those most likely to be affected. These are also the causes. So too are many factors which affect the way we bring up our children; as Sir Keith says, "when a child is deprived of constant love and guidance he is deprived of that background most likely to lead to stability and maturity ... Nobody's asking people to be ideal parents, just good enough parents".'
> (4.6.1973)

Typical in this passage is the way in which emotional disorder and economic causation are jumbled together so that both equally become part of the inadequacy of the individual. The very use of the popular word 'deprivation' facilitates this muddle. What is interesting is to find these ideas taken up by a senior Government Minister and translated into policy in the shape of the Family Income Supplement and of research projects. FIS is a means tested benefit which heads of families, provided they are men, in employment may claim so long as their wage does not come above a certain level. It is therefore a social security benefit which, like Speenhamland, both supports very low wage levels and bolsters up the family. The DHSS also commissioned the Social Science Research Council to undertake a large scale scheme of research into the 'Cycle' and in 1974 a preliminary statement, *The Needs of Children* (1974) by Mia Kellmer Pringle, Director of the National Children's Bureau, appeared, intended as a 'source document' for work to be done on planning for parenthood and the Cycle of Deprivation generally. Mia Kellmer Pringle has presented herself as a 'radical' thinker so far as child-rearing is concerned, and has led a new trend (embodied in the 1975 *Children Act*) which has moved away from an interpretation of Bowlby that views the best place for the child as being always with its parents, and towards a view that, implying even more exalted standards of child care, judges certain parents as being unfit to look after their children. In practice, some children have always had to be removed from their parents, but only as a last resort; the new thinking interprets the reception of children into care in a new, more 'positive' light without confronting the question of who it is that decides, and by what criteria, which parents are unfit. Mia Kellmer Pringle does not question the superiority of middle-class standards of child rearing; she does not recognize how the constraints of economic hardship and poor housing may actually prevent parents from fulfilling their own standards of child care; nor does she recognize changing demographic trends which surely reflect what men and women want in the way of family life. In an article in *The Times* (14.1.1976) Mia Kellmer Pringle spelt out her 'scenario for the future' – 'revolutionary' ideas which turn out to be extraordinarily similar to those put forward by Edith Summerskill (*see* Hopkinson 1971 : 145–48) in 1945. Going directly against population trends which show that while more individual women (and men) are choosing to become parents, fewer wish to devote their whole lives to it, she makes the old suggestion of motherhood as a paid career, with those women who are specially fitted for it taking it on in a new spirit: 'Mothering should be recognized as the important, skilled and demanding job it is. . . . Hence, adequate financial reward must be provided so that no mother of under-fives has to go out to work for financial reasons. Husbands should have to acknowledge the value of looking after young families by sharing their income with their wives as of right. Also the state should pay a salary to mothers.' The rest should eschew motherhood: 'Women's, and indeed men's, right to choose or reject parenthood for themselves must be conceded unquestioningly and without any implied reproach.'

Journalists (e.g. Crabtree in *The Guardian* 22.1.1976) too, are climbing on the band wagon and blaming parental greed if the

mother works. Yet usually mothers work from financial necessity, and Kellmer Pringle does not confront the economic consequences of her suggestions. She makes one further suggestion,
for the 'radical alternative' of shared parenthood, which, if fully
shared:

> 'would mean rotating the [home-making] role, each parent in
> turn undertaking it for say a [three or four] year period. The
> mother would probably opt for [the child's early] care to con-
> solidate the initial bonds cre[ated at birth. Employers] may
> cavil at the idea of a rotatin[g male/female work force.] Yet
> many occupations lend thems[elves quite readily to such inter-]
> changeability ... Those who [opt for a life-style of shared]
> parenthood will have to cho[ose a like-minded partner. This]
> may well ensure a more dura[ble and satisfying union.]
>
> *(The Times* 14.1.1976)

Such marriages do occur i[n, for example, Sw]eden, yet while
theoretically practicable, [it implies the high] valuation of an
intensely inturned ar[d symbiotic couple] relationship. Many
British and Wester[n European marri]ages are very family
and couple centred [already, and it is] generally believed (e.g.
Fletcher 1963) that [higher divorc]e and marriage breakdown
rates have come a[bout more ...] for this reason – that so great
an emotional in[vestment is made] in a single relationship. On the
other hand, [is there any] logical reason why Dr Kellmer
Pringle conf[ines the shared]-parenthood 'life-style' to a monogamous co[uple? Why not] extend it to group marriage?

At the [same time oth]er theoreticians have approached the
proble[ms and future] of family life from another perspective.
Marg[aret Wynn,] for example, has consciously confronted
the t[ask of ensuring the] best possible development of 'human
capi[tal' in the n]ext generation of workers, and to back her
ar[gument she qu]otes the *Newsom Report* which frankly stated
[that what is nee]d is ... for a generally better educated and in-
[creasingly ad]aptable labour force to meet new demands.' She
[points out that at any g]iven time only about twenty-two per
[cent of the population ar]e engaged in the rearing of children, but
[this small perc]entage bears almost the whole cost. Her
solution is for the State to share in this, mainly by increasing
family allowances according to the age of the child; and for

tax and other benefits to be redistributed towards families with children. This more sophisticated version of selectivity is known as 'positive discrimination' but would only be truly progressive were it to involve a redistribution of wealth along class lines as well. The kind of redistribution suggested by Margaret Wynn, however, is only lateral – from non-parents to parents. Nevertheless, the widespread discussion of various forms of income support specifically for families in recent years, another example of which would be the debate aroused by the Tory proposals for a Tax Credit (1972) system, demonstrates increased concern as well as the worsening economic situation.

Social policy proposals have consistently sought to support both the economic system and the institution of the family. Bill Jordan (1974) has raised the vital question whether these two goals are mutually compatible. In a criticism of the Cycle of Deprivation theory he has pointed out that many of the traits said to be associated with poverty – helplessness, inadequacy, passive lethargy, living for the moment – are self-preservative within our welfare system, which does not in practice always support the family unit. For instance, in some circumstances a woman with children may be better off drawing social security than depending on a man, if he is earning very low wages, or if he is unemployed and attempts are being made to pressure him into taking work; a woman alone is more likely for one thing to be awarded exceptional needs grants. Jordan himself however, although he takes a radical standpoint, completely fails to come to grips with the central problem facing not only women but society: child care. He criticizes women for demanding paid work, which he regards as even more alienated than the role of housewife, and he accepts, quoting Simon Yudkin and Anthea Holme (1963), that children below the age of three should not be separated from their mothers at all, and presumably he would agree with Mia Kellmer Pringle that 'In western societies, no wholly adequate substitute has been found for the one-to-one, close, continuing, loving and mutually enjoyable relationship which is the hall-mark of maternal care' (*The Times* 14.1.1976). This is itself a re-statement of Bowlby's beliefs, and a re-examination of Bowlby's writings reveals as rather odd his stress exclusively on the maternal role. In his cult of the mother–

baby relationship Bowlby, as Elsa Ferri (1976) has recently pointed out, saw the father as : 'of no direct importance to the young child but (he) is of indirect value as an economic support and in his emotional support of the mother'. And in his more recent work (1969) Bowlby has taken this even further and sought to prove by means of comparisons with tribal societies and with subhuman primates that the 'natural' social formation is the mother and her brood of children – possibly supported by her own mother and the mother's younger children – rather than the nuclear family inclusive of the father. A number of writers (Andry 1971; Bronfenbrenner 1970; Comfort 1970) have challenged this view, as it happens, but only in so far as a more important role for the father is both desirable and also is actually the case. Michael Rutter (1972) has demonstrated conclusively the questionable nature of Bowlby's work and the many areas where we are still above all *ignorant* of the causation and meaning of 'attachment behaviour' in children, and hence too in adults. What needs to be explained is the strength of society's attachment to Bowlby's theories and the effect this has had on social policies which have since the war operated on an unquestioning assumption of the unique and irreplaceable nature of the mother–child bond. This has had a repressive effect on the lives of women in two distinct ways. First, the reality that many women become deeply depressed when confined in an isolated way to the home with small children (see Brown, Sklair, Harris and Birley 1973a, 1973b; Brown 1974; Brown, Ní Bholcháiri, and Harris 1975; Brown, Harris, and Copeland 1976; Brown 1976) has been ignored, and secondly Bowlby has been an excuse for failure to provide alternative forms of care for children, and has even inhibited creative thought on the subject. The few State nursery places continue to be reserved for unsupported parents and baby batterers, that is for deviants. Indeed the *Finer Report*, for all its liberalism accepted Bowlby unthinkingly and presents a view of the one-parent family as essentially a mutilated form of the 'normal' family. Its recommendations aim to remove the economic disabilities of one-parent families only within the structure of present family relationships.

SIX

Welfare in the twentieth century

I shall now look backwards over the development of twentieth century welfare legislation to try to trace how anti-feminism became so entrenched within our social policies before discussing finally, how the present situation offers possibilities for change in both a reactionary and a progressive direction.

During the nineteenth century the public health movement (Finer 1952) had represented an effort by the Victorians to deal with the diswelfares brought about by the urbanization consequent upon industrialization, while the *Factory Acts* and the *Poor Law* had primarily been attempts to deal with problems of employment and the labour market. Out of these however, by reason of the educational provisions for the young embodied in the *Factory Acts*, and by reason of the kinds of individuals to be found in Poor Law institutions, had gradually emerged a new and more complex understanding of the nature and extent of poverty and destitution. In the 1880s, when the Victorian fear of the revolutionary menace of the poor, especially the poor of London's East End, was at its height there began also to be an increasing concern with poverty, and a new awareness that it was not invariably the fault of the poor themselves. Writing in 1913, Alfred Spender, editor of the *Westminster Gazette* described this change in consciousness:

> ' "It is difficult after thirty years to realise the shock of novelty with which revelations of the condition of the poor came to comfortable people in the seventies or eighties, or the sensation which such a pamphlet as *The Bitter Cry of Outcast London* made when it was first produced. The separateness of the poor life and the rich life had hardened to a point at which mutual ignorance and repudiation of responsibility threatened to become fixed in English thought. Social legislation was declared to be outside the sphere of Parliament and most philanthropic schemes were denounced as pauperising the poor. [Canon] Barnett's effort was to break down this separation of classes and enlarge the idea of social responsibility." '
> (Barnett 1919:309)

The 'New Philanthropy' also recognized that, now they had the vote, working men had the power to alter the conditions under which they lived (see Gilbert 1966:25–6) and so gradually new and more highly differentiated forms of positive welfare intervention began to be introduced. In 1885 the rigours of the Poor Law were softened by an Amendment, the *Medical Relief (Disqualification Removal) Act*, which allowed a citizen to receive medical attention without becoming officially a pauper and being disenfranchised, and later came the *Outdoor Relief (Friendly Societies) Act* of 1894 which allowed a small disregarded sum of Friendly Society savings to relief applicants. Then the immediate result of the Trafalgar Square riot was Joseph Chamberlain's Government Board circular, which encouraged local authorities to set up public works to relieve unemployment, and showed that government now recognized the social nature of unemployment and the appropriateness of state intervention.

(Another consequence of the riot was the beginning of private labour exchanges.) These changes and innovations, small in themselves, suggest that the poor were beginning to be perceived no longer 'in a lump' but as individuals with varying needs and, often, disabilities, for it was already known (see Pinker 1971) that the majority of inmates of workhouses were not the able-bodied poor (supposedly the work-shy), but orphans, the sick, and the aged infirm. Henceforth, and increasingly in the twentieth century, social policy was to embrace the two distinct yet related areas of employment on the one hand and the care of the non-working members of the population on the other, and from this it was a natural development for the State to try to promote, with what is known as positive legislation, the kind of society thought to be desirable, by means of its welfare provisions.

Yet even as the horrors of outcast London (Stedman Jones 1971) were being revealed to polite society, legislation and innovations such as cheap transport and workmen's fares were acting to change the situation with the dispersal of the more respectable working-class families from the slums to new working-class suburbs in East and South London, and the 1880s saw both the culmination of fears of the revolutionary potential of the workless hordes, and their passing. Notwithstanding the upsurge of left-wing political activity within the working class during the closing years of the century, and the widespread political disturbances of the Edwardian era (Dangerfield 1971) the new Social Imperialist position which developed perceived the questions of poverty and unemployment more in relation to imperial effectiveness and national strength than in relation to internal disorder and unrest. This period of rapid imperialist expansion (Cole and Postgate 1961) was reflected in the development of an imperialist consciousness, and the mission of the ruling class and their representatives – civil servants, teachers, the students from the universities who made up the strength of the Settlement Movement – was literally seen as being to bring a more civilized way of life not only to the pigmies and cannibals of Africa and the Hindus of India, but also to the drunks, prostitutes, and degenerates of the Metropolis itself. The literature of the Settlement Movement (Simon (1965) contains good material on the Settlement Movement) is full of such aspirations, expressed with a naive optimism in the superiority of civilized British life. It is easy to see how positive welfare legislation could fit very well into this view of the world.

Even before the 1899 recruiting drive for the Boer War had revealed the facts to the public at large, the physical puniness and general ill health and debility of the British worker had been known to the authorities. Wider discussion, however, in terms of the country's fitness to fulfil her imperial role overseas led to an Interdepartmental Committee on Physical Deterioration, set up in 1903, and its Report, published the following year, made various recommendations which formed the basis for some of the Liberal legislation of the 1906 to 1911 years. It recommended that the State should consider the extension and enforcement of regulations over environmental health conditions; the enforcement and extension of building and sanitary regulations in factories and homes and control of the distribution of food and handling of milk. Particularly significant in the context of women's role were its recommendations that mothers should be taught proper child care and girls should be taught cookery and dietetics; and it also recommended that there should be curbs on adult drinking and juvenile smoking; that the State should make an effort to encourage physical training and exercise; that there should be proper school medical inspections; and finally that there should be a State sponsored system for the feeding of school children.

A second reason for the concern surrounding the aspiration towards national efficiency was the fact of the declining birthrate. During the last quarter of the nineteenth century the size of families had begun to decline, from thirty-five live births per thousand of the population in the 1870s to twenty-five per thousand in 1910 (Banks and Banks 1964), a process which had begun in the middle classes (although there is evidence (Hewitt 1958) that birth control was also at this time being practised by certain sections of the working class). A new consciousness amongst women mean that the hitherto endless cycle of pregnancy, birth, and infant care no longer seemed inevitable. Women themselves had not necessarily enjoyed or accepted this necessary part of their sacred vocation as mother. Queen Victoria herself had complained about it (Fulford 1964) and, many years later, Flora Thompson recorded the reaction of her mother, a working-class countrywoman:

'[My mother] lived to see the decline in the birth rate, and, when she discussed it with [me] in the early 1930s, laughed heartily at some of the explanations advanced by the learned, and said: "If they knew what it meant to carry and bear and and bring up a child themselves, they wouldn't expect the women to be in a hurry to have a second or third now they've got a say in the matter.' (Thompson 1973:429–30)

The Fabians who were ardent advocates of national efficiency and took up an imperialist position expressed a preoccupation with eugenics that was widely prevalent throughout society and greatly influenced social science. Sidney Ball for example wrote:

'The socialist policy, so far from favouring the weak, favours the strong ... it is a process of conscious social selection by which the industrial residuum is naturally sifted and made manageable for some kind of restorative, disciplinary, or, it may be, "surgical" treatment ... In this way it not only favours the growth of the fittest within the group, but also the fittest group in the world competition of societies.'
(Ball 1896)

and William Beveridge, who was not a Fabian but who at this period was close to the Webbs expressed similar sentiments:

' "The ideal should *not* be an industrial system arranged with a view to finding room in it for everyone who desired to enter, but an industrial system in which everyone who *did* find a place at all should obtain average earnings at least up to the standard of healthy subsistence ... The line between independence and dependence, between the efficient and the unemployable has to be made clearer and broader ... those men who through general defects are unable to fill such a whole place in industry are to be recognised as unemployable. They must become the acknowledged dependants of the State, removed from free industry and maintained adequately in public institutions, but with a complete and permanent loss of all citizen rights including not only the franchise, but civil freedom and fatherhood." ' (Stedman Jones 1971:334)

This rather sinister preoccupation with eugenics seems closer to national socialism than to any other kind; H. G. Wells and Arnold White (1901) did openly advocate the sterilization of the unfit. But the fear of national degeneration was heightened because it was believed that the poor were breeding at a much faster rate than the rest of the population. The solution put forward by Sidney Webb and others was not implementation of the recommendations of the Interdepartmental Committee, but State action to encourage the wealthier sections of society to reproduce themselves. In the Fabian tract *The Decline of the Birthrate* (1907) Sidney Webb called for a 'revolution in the economic incidence of child-bearing' and for the 'endowment of motherhood', that is State pensions for mothers.

Thirdly, with a new mass of working-class voters it was natural that social reform began to be consciously used as an alternative to, and bulwark against, socialism, particularly during the years of industrial militancy (Halévy 1934) before the First World War. Lloyd George, Winston Churchill, and William Beveridge were all well aware of the reforms introduced by Bismarck's authoritarian imperialist administration in Germany. Both Lloyd George and Beveridge visited Germany and returned more determined than ever to set up similar schemes in this country. Later W. J. Braithwaite (Bunbury 1957) was sent to have a more detailed look at the German scheme. The result was a form of State national insurance scheme which, Bentley Gilbert (1966) has suggested, represented a step into a new and uncharted field. He has described the *Unemployed Workmen Act* of 1905, brought in by a Conservative government, as the last in a line of attempts to deal with the results of unemployment by the remedy of relief work. A new approach was inaugurated four years later with the 1909 *Labour Exchanges Act*. Labour exchanges were Beveridge's answer to the problem of unemployment (Beveridge 1909). (They were later to facilitate the organization of labour during the War (Hinton 1973).) He, like the Webbs, tended to perceive unemployment as a problem to be dealt with by rationalization of the labour market without fully appreciating the extent to which jobs might actually not be available even for those who were most sincerely seeking work. It is in this context of a more hesitant and less dogmatic attitude towards unemployment that the Royal Commission on the Poor Law (1905–1909) should be seen. Set up by the Conservatives as a result of considerable debate surrounding the 1905 *Unemployed Workmen Act*, it split and eventually produced both a Majority and a Minority Report. Both recognized implicitly the shortcomings of the *Poor Law* as it then existed, but only the Minority Report (largely the work of the Webbs) recommended its complete break up. They believed that in the interests of efficiency its various responsibilities for the sick, the old, and children should be distributed to specialist departments. The Minority Report also recognized prevention as the only way to cope with destitution; a proper minimum of subsistence should be assured to those who needed it. In fact two assumptions underlay the Report. One was a sociological rather than a socialist approach to the nature of poverty. This was not seen as a unifying force, but as rising from a diversity of causes which needed to be examined, understood, and eliminated. Ironically this assumption has become embedded in modern social work, although the Webbs themselves saw no place for social workers in the society they desired to bring about. Their second assumption was that State support should imply a mutual obligation; the recipient of a service should pay for it if he had the means, if not, the provision of a service should involve the obligation of the recipient to co-operate in 'treatment' for his condition; thus the Webbs believed that the unemployed should be compelled if necessary to move to new employment or a labour colony, and that the provision of help should be given only on the undertaking of reformation by the idler or criminal. Training schemes, like medical treatment, should be compulsory.

The Majority Report was based on no such clear ideological set of assumptions, and suggested modifications rather than the complete break up of the *Poor Law*. As Helen Bosanquet admits, the various members of the COS, while they supported the Majority Report, did not feel that it properly reflected the views of their organization, and she gives the impression that they were finding it hard at this time to come to terms with the shocking facts of poverty and destitution revealed by the evidence presented to the Commission.

The Reports did in ·fact confirm both the more sensational findings of writers like Andrew Mearns, and the scientific research of Charles Booth and softened public opinion so that social provision became more acceptable. Because the Commission split, it was all the easier for the Liberal Government to take no direct action in attacking the *Poor Law* – which would still have been a highly controversial step to take – and its reforms in fact by-passed the whole issue. Lloyd George himself did recognize that the *1911 Insurance Act* was a political substitute for what the Minority Report in particular had envisaged, a complete reorganization of welfare services within a positive welfare framework and he wrote:

> ' "Insurance necessary temporary expedient. At no distant date hope State will acknowledge a full responsibility in the matter of making provision for sickness, breakdown and unemployment. It really does so now, through Poor Law, but conditions under which this system had hitherto worked have been so harsh and humiliating that working class pride revolts against accepting so degrading and doubtful a boon." '
>
> (M. E. Rose 1972:50)

Far from being a temporary expedient however, the insurance principle has become enshrined in our welfare system. Richard Titmuss has criticized both Reports and suggested that the type of concern being expressed and the kinds of reform later instituted were still suffused with the old nineteenth century beliefs about the behaviour of the individual, which saw social problems in terms of symptoms instead of in terms of underlying causation, whether social or psychological. Thus an over-simplified utilitarian model of economic man has been preserved in a fossilized state in much twentieth century welfare legislation, and still stamps it to this day.

The *National Insurance Act* was nonetheless an important measure. Although it covered only a low-risk group of skilled workers, $2\frac{1}{4}$ million out of a possible 10 million (and hardly any women at all), it was significant in that it married conscious State intervention in the manner of Germany, to the insurance ideal as it had existed in Victorian England in the shape of Friendly Societies, trades union schemes, and commercial insurance, and tried to perpetuate the ideal of self-help and independence (as the *Beveridge Report* was later to do). Nonetheless, the scheme was by no means wholeheartedly welcomed by the Labour Movement, who suspected a concealed attack on wages; in addition many trades unions disliked it precisely because they had schemes of their own. National health insurance likewise represented a compromise between conflicting interests and Emmeline Pethick Lawrence was one woman who foresaw that it would be the interests of women that would be sacrificed to the powerful unions and still more powerful commercial insurance companies:

' "Instead of providing that a weekly allowance of five shillings should be paid to every widow having a child or children under sixteen years of age and that a weekly allowance of five shillings should be paid to the man in sickness as agreed by the friendly societies, Mr Lloyd George struck the widow out of the Bill altogether and instead of giving five shillings to the man ... gave ten shillings to the man and nothing to the widow. It was done because Mr Lloyd George had to make his bill as attractive as possible to the working man, especially the aristocracy of labour in this country and he thought it would be a better bribe, a draw for the working man if he increased the insurance of the man and withdrew the insurance of the widow." '   (Gilbert 1966:331)

All in all, the Act well illustrates what Bentley Gilbert commented upon as 'the curious opposing pressures to which social legislation seems to be particularly vulnerable'. (The *Old Age Pension Act* of 1908 although it also represented only a very partial solution to the poverty of old age was the only measure to be welcomed wholeheartedly by the people themselves, perhaps because it was at first non-contributory, although there was a moral element in the sense that pensions were supposed to be withheld from those 'who had habitually failed to work according to ability and need and those who had failed to save money regularly'.)

Whereas the National Insurance scheme was clearly an attempt to provide State assistance in a context that managed to retain an emphasis on individualism (the individual worker insuring himself and his family by means of a contribution from his own wage), Old Age Pensions did represent the fulfilment of a demand from the workers themselves, and there had been for a number of years a National Committee of Organised Labour for Promoting Old Age Pensions. The provision of school meals for children was also a measure for which progressive reformers and the labour movement struggled for many years.

France had pioneered in this field but in this country, too, there had long been an awareness of the problem of the under-nourished children of the poor, first noticed when the ragged schools were set up, but here there were more strenuous attempts than on the Continent to deal with it by voluntary, charitable means. In 1864 the Destitute Children's Dinner Society was set up and, operating on COS lines, it was hoped that the dinners provided could be made to pay for themselves, the parents paying a penny for the meal. In practice however it was difficult to enforce payment, especially when, as the School Board Chronicle of 1884 commented:

' "We must not teach poor children or poor parents to lean upon Charity, but on the other hand, it ought never to be forgotten that this new law of compulsory attendance at school, in the making whereof the poorest classses of the people had no hand whatever exacts greater sacrifices from that class than from any other ... The very poor ... never asked to have education provided for their children, never wanted it, have practically nothing to gain by it and much to lose, and ... this law of compulsory education is forced on them not for their good or for their pleasure, but for the safety and progress of society and for the sake of economy in the administration of the laws in the matter of Poor Relief and Crime." '
(Bulkley 1914:11–12)

Because of the chaos and variability of provision of meals a special committee was appointed in 1889 and its report showed that whereas in some districts dinners were provided wastefully and to children who did not need them, in others children were virtually starving, or were fed only once or twice a week. It was calculated that 43,888 or 12¾ per cent of the children attending Board Schools were habitually in want of food, and of these less than half were being provided for. The Committee therefore recommended a rationalization and centralization of provision and as a result the London Schools Dinner Association was founded. Provision of dinners was everywhere for 'needy' children only, and this had the result that schools meals were tainted with the notion of charity, and there was always an assumption that it was 'better' if children ate at home, and a negative comment on a mother if she was unable to feed her own children. As has often happened, rich and poor concurred in their condemnation of the mother who relied on welfare, and on the poor mother as an inadequate mother. These themes are persistent ones in the history of welfare.

In 1905 there was an attempt to make the *Poor Law* feed necessitous children, and its failure to do this was part of a general discrediting of the *Poor Law*. The attempt did however establish a precedent for State intervention, although many parents withdrew their children for fear of being designated paupers. At the same time thousands of children whose parents were not technically destitute, simply very badly paid, lost their right to the meals they needed. This further revealed the general inadequacies of Poor Law provision and showed how necessary school meals were, since, as the Hammersmith Guardians themselves commented:

' "When school children's parents are in receipt of outdoor relief, that fact should be taken as an indication that such children would be benefitted by school meals and not as an indication that they are adequately fed, since as a matter of fact outdoor relief is seldom or never adequate." '

(Bulkley 1914:165)

Finally came the *Education (Feeding of School Children) Act* of 1906. Although largely permissive it caused outcry, particularly because of the paragraph stipulating that notwithstanding any failure by parents to pay for the meals provided for their children, these parents were to suffer no loss of civil rights or privileges – meals were in the last analysis to be provided free. Thus was established the principle of State intervention with a positive end in mind. Opposition to it too was on this basis, and, for instance, Margaret McMillan, campaigning for school meals in Bradford (a town which became a pioneer in the field) found herself opposed by the Liberal majority on the Council for precisely this reason – that the provision of the midday meal would reduce parental authority and responsibility. A. V. Dicey saw in the Act the beginning of the slide towards socialism that culminated in national insurance and argued that the privileges of citizenship implied the successful fulfilment of the individual's private and family obligations – 'Why a man who first neglects his duty as a father and then defrauds the State should retain his full political rights is a question easier to ask than to answer' (Gilbert 1966:113). As the provision of meals remained very variable throughout the country, a second *Education (Provision of Meals) Act* in 1914 established school meals as a compulsory obligation of local government. Even more important, school medical officers were henceforth to be the sole judges of which children were to be fed, and this finally removed the whole issue from the arena of the Poor Law and made it a question of physical condition and the facilitation of learning.

Other measures to promote the health of mothers and children met with none of the ideological opposition to which the provision of school meals was subjected; infant mortality was attacked with legislation to provide free milk for babies, and the beginnings of the health-visiting and midwifery services were inaugurated. There was also the beginning of school medical inspections in 1907. These were seen as an effort to facilitate education, rather than being a direct, crude response to the *Physical Deterioration Committee Report*. In Bradford they were being carried out before that Report, and Margaret McMillan and other progressives who campaigned for this Act saw it in terms of providing medical treatment, not just inspection – since the problem that medical inspection brought was how the necessary treatment was to be carried out, for in most cases the only medical treatment provided free was under the *Poor Law* which again made those receiving it technically paupers. Like so many welfare measures, therefore, school medical inspection did raise further issues, but although again, it was discussed in terms of national efficiency, it should also be seen as part of a generally heightened consciousness of child care, hygiene, and medicine. Finally the *1908 Children's Act* was a consolidating measure which brought together earlier scattered legislation relating to infant life protection and was extended to cover parental neglect. This too was a significant inroad into the principle of parental rights and of the child as the property of his father, yet it too became law without controversy.

These measures all represent, in part, the imperialist response to the falling birthrate and the alleged physical degeneration of the masses. They were measures intended at one and the same time to bring the poverty stricken hordes within the pale of British civilization and to make possible a rising generation of men fit to shoulder the white man's burden and women fit to bear their sons. We should feel no surprise that these pre-occupations should have included an intensified consciousness of the need to promote motherhood by means of positive legislation, guidance, and control. General William Booth in his popular book *In Darkest England and the Way Out* typified such an attitude:

> 'Take the girls. Who can pretend that the girls our schools are now turning out are half as well educated for the work of life as their grandmothers were at the same age? How many of these mothers of the future know how to bake a loaf or wash their clothes? Except minding the baby – a task that cannot be evaded – what domestic training have they received to qualify them for being in the future the mothers of babies themselves? ... The home is largely destroyed where the mother follows the father into the factory, and where the hours of labour are so long that they have not time to see their children ... It is the home that has been destroyed, and with the home the home-like virtues. It is the dis-homed multitude, nomadic, hungry, that is rearing an undisciplined population, cursed from birth with hereditary weakness of body and hereditary faults of character ... Nothing is worth doing ... that does not Reconstitute the Home.'
> (Booth 1890:65–6)

Similarly General John Frederick Maurice, writing in the *Contemporary Review* in 1902 drew on the observations of Canon Barnett who had pointed out that the Jewish women in Whitechapel – living in the same appalling slum conditions as Englishwomen there – enjoyed a greater life expectancy. This was attributed to the one difference between them, that the Gentile women went out to work and the Jewish women did not. (There was also a widespread feeling that the employment of children was unhealthy.) Louisa Twining in her autobiography (1893) described how working-class mothers were being taught to carry out their role:

'A method now largely carried out by mothers' meetings and unions, as well as by the excellent teaching given in lectures and pamphlets of the National Health Society and Ladies Sanitary Association, and also, I must add, by the admirable personal influence of the many district nurses who are now importing sound instruction, not only with regard to sickness but in sanitary and preventive measures as well.'

(Twining 1893 : 160)

At the same time, social workers were ceasing to be voluntary workers and were becoming professionalized. By 1892 Octavia Hill was planning the training of her workers and seeing the Southwark University Women's Settlement as a natural centre for this. The first university course for social workers opened at the London School of Economics in 1912.

The type of woman likely to take up social work and social administration in the Edwardian period was different from her Victorian sisters, yet different also from the 'new woman' of whom Ibsen, Shaw, and H. G. Wells wrote. There was then, as there is now, a tendency (no more than that) for the emancipation of women to be seen in two distinct ways. There were those women who demanded new social freedoms. Anne Veronica, H. G. Wells's emancipated heroine (something of a caricature) decided that her place was not with the Suffragettes since she wanted to give herself more fully to men, finding sexual fulfilment and 'freedom' in a new kind of submission. Cristabel Pankhurst might preach chastity and total withdrawal from men, but many of the young women of the nineties demanded that they be allowed to smoke, to travel alone, and to see men by themselves, free from the surveillance of the chaperone. Even the right to sexual experience was no longer a thing completely unheard of. As early as 1881 Frances Power Cobbe had warned of the dangers, as she saw them, of these new customs:

'It was almost my foremost object to do all that might be possible for me to separate the sacred cause of the social and political emancipation of women from certain modes of thought and action which it has been the business of false friends and open enemies to confound these with. The preachers of the hateful and disgusting doctrines of free love have been the bane and calamity of our allies in America. We have nothing quite so bad here; but we have, in the highest circles, a new development of "fastness" very nearly akin to profligacy and quite akin to the neglect of all decorum and womanly dignity; and we have in the middle class also a new tone, if not of behaviour yet of opinion; a tone of laxity in discussing breaches of the law of chastity which must prove no less disastrous in its results than it is, in my opinion, erroneous in principle.'   (Power Cobbe 1881 : 132)

By the time Edward VII ascended the throne bicycling and tennis had made girls healthier and more energetic as well as widening their social horizons and giving them more freedom from the restrictions of stifling clothes as well as stifling conventions; in more bohemian circles it was possible for a young woman like Katherine Mansfield to live an unsupervised life and take a lover without courting the social ostracism and perhaps sexual degradation that she might once have risked (although the fate of the Victorian kept woman was not always as dark as the Victorian myth would have had contemporaries believe (Basch 1974)).

The Suffragettes on the other hand tended to preach sexual restraint for both sexes as an alternative to the double standard which was the norm, and many of the more progressive young women of the period shared this view. Beatrice Webb for example, held to the then rather widely prevalent belief in a moral distinction between men and women, and her comment on Henrietta Barnett suggests the importance of this frame of reference for the development of women's work :

'Her personal aim in life is to raise womanhood to its rightful position; as equal though unlike manhood. The crusade she has undertaken is the fight against impurity as the main factor in debasing women from a status of independence to one of physical dependence ... I told her that the only way in which we can convince the world of our power is to show it. And for that it will be needful for women with strong natures to remain celibate; so that the special force of womanhood – motherly feeling – may be forced into public work.'   (Webb 1969 : 223)

It was significant for the development of welfare work that the women who interested themselves in it were likely to come from precisely that high-minded and earnest section of bourgeois society that tended to minimize women's sexuality and to pose public work as an alternative to family life. Beatrice Webb made a further interesting comment on a plan of Octavia Hill's to attract 'stronger and finer' women into the profession that was to become social work:

> '*I* believe in the attraction of belonging to a *body* who have a definite mission and a definite expression, and where the stronger and more ambitious natures rise and lead. I admire and reverence women most who are content to be among the "unknown saints". But it is no use shutting one's eyes to the fact that there is an increasing number of women to whom a matrimonial career is shut, and who seek a masculine reward for masculine qualities. There is in these women something exceedingly pathetic, and I would do anything to open careers to them in which their somewhat abnormal but useful qualities would get their own reward ... I think these strong women have a great future before them in the solution of social questions. They are not just inferior men; they may have masculine faculty; but they have the woman's temperament, and the stronger they are the more distinctively feminine they are in this. I hope that, instead of trying to ape men and take up men's pursuits, they will carve out their own careers, and not be satisfied until they have found the careers in which their particular form of power will achieve most.'   (Webb 1969:281)

(The equal but different argument was used on both sides in the debate about the suffrage. Octavia Hill (Moberley Bell 1942), for example used it to argue against women having the vote.)

Between these and the working-class women to whom they ministered a great gulf remained fixed. Even with the beginnings of a wider use of birth-control, working-class families especially remained large:

> 'The typical working-class mother of the 1890s, married in her teens or early twenties and experiencing ten pregnancies, spent about fifteen years in a state of pregnancy

and in nursing a child for the first year of its life. She was tied, for this period of time, to the wheel of childbearing. Today, for the typical mother, the time so spent would be about four years ...

At the beginning of this century, the expectation of life of a woman aged twenty was forty-six years. Approximately one third of this life expectancy was to be devoted to the physiological and emotional experiences of childbearing and maternal care in infancy. Today, the expectation of life of a woman aged twenty is fifty-five years. Of this longer expectation only about seven per cent of the years to be lived will be concerned with childbearing and maternal care in infancy.'

(Titmuss 1963:91)

Seebohm Rowntree commented more graphically on the monotony of the lives of working-class women:

'Probably this monotony is least marked in the slum districts, where life is lived more in common, and where the women are constantly in and out of each other's houses, or meet and gossip in the courts and streets. But with advance in the social scale, family life becomes more private, and the women, left in the house all day whilst their husbands are at work, are largely thrown upon their own resources ... These women too often become mere hopeless drudges ... The husband commonly finds his chief interest among his "mates" and seldom rises even to the idea of mental companionship. He rarely illtreats her; but restricted education and a narrow circle of activities hinder comradeship, and lack of mental touch tends to pass into unconscious neglect or active selfishness. It must be remembered too, that we are dealing with a class who do not keep domestic servants. The mother of a young family is not therefore able to escape from her circumstances through the cultivation of those social amenities which are the relief of her wealthier sisters. Even when able to get away for a day's holiday, or to go out for the evening, she is often obliged to take a baby with her. It is plain therefore that the conditions which govern the life of the women are gravely unsatisfactory, and are the more serious in their consequences since the character and attractive power of the family life are principally dependent upon her.'   (Seebohm Rowntree 1901 : 108–9)

In general, the remedy was seen in the elimination of poverty and in a more positive promotion of happy child care. Even Margaret McMillan in her pioneering work to promote nursery school education saw this as drawing mothers in so that they should take a new interest in their children's development (see McMillan 1919; Lowndes 1960).

Socialists generally continued confused as to the relationship between family and State. Mrs Ramsay MacDonald for example:

'considered the essential function of Socialism to be the protection of the home. J. Ramsey MacDonald writes : "She once defined Socialism as the State of Homes" and he himself stated in 1908 : "Socialism is essential to family life ... the idea of divorce is foreign to the Socialist State." '

(Halévy 1934 : 510)

Some ILP leaders were openly hostile to the WSPU, the militant suffragettes. Nor did the Suffragettes themselves challenge the ideal of woman as Mother, although by their deeds they did implicitly challenge the prevailing views of ladylike behaviour, so that it is perhaps not surprising that when they left their drawing rooms and rose up in revolt against patriarchal society they met with execration and horror (Pankhurst 1911, 1931; Rosen 1974; Ramelson 1965), for they dared to expose the sex antagonism underlying the politenesses of Edwardian society.

The Suffragettes married a constitutional demand with the tactics of revolutionary violence. Their gut feminism had a feeling for something that was wrong with sexual, if not with family, relationships, yet it could not attack the idealization of Motherhood, for it had no worked-out analysis of the position of women; nor could it meet the working-class and labour movement strength, which co-existed with an entirely bourgeois approach to the family and women's role. The revolt of the women was ultimately inchoate; the labour movement was drawn towards reformism. Between the two the State slipped in and started to build a cage for the working-class family.

After the First World War women were granted the vote, but how they were really valued was more clearly to be judged from the speed with which they were ejected from the labour market:

'The end of the war brought the financial prosperity of women to a sudden stop. No later than the spring of 1919 the demobilisation of women war-workers was in full swing, and the most miserable consequences were following from it ... Thousands upon thousands of women workers were dismissed and found no work to do. It was difficult to see how this could have been prevented. All the special war work was at an end, industry was contracting and not expanding, and such jobs as there were had to be kept for the returning soldiers. This was the governing factor, and nothing could change it; and yet it was terribly hard on the women. Everyone assumed of course that they would go quietly back to their homes, and that everything could be as it had been before, but apart altogether from anything the women might wish this was sheerly impossible. The war had enormously increased the number of surplus women so that very nearly one in three had to be self-supporting; it had broken up innumerable homes and brought into existence a great class of new poor. Prices were nearly double what they had been in 1914 and the women who had been able to live on their small fixed allowances or fixed incomes could do so no more. All these facts were however forgotten. Public opinion assumed that all women could still be supported by men, and that if they went on working it was from a sort of deliberate wickedness. The tone of the Press swung, all in a moment, from extravagant praise to the opposite extreme and the very same people who had become heroines and saviours of their country a few months before were now parasites, blacklegs and limpets. Employers were implored to turn them out as passionately as they had been implored to employ them and their last weeks in their wartime jobs were made miserable by the jeers and taunts of their fellow workers. The women themselves acquiesced in the situation.'

(Strachey 1928:370–71)

It had been feared that when women got the vote some kind of

Women's Party might be formed and women might vote as a bloc. This did not happen, so there was little opposition to the extension of the vote to women over twenty-one (the Flapper vote) in 1928. The very few women MPs inevitably were drawn into a position where their special task seemed to be to speak for women and to concern themselves with 'women's problems' within Parliament; prices, social policy, and domestic matters were their sphere. Many feminists assumed that 'the main fight is over and the main victory is won' (Strachey 1928) and turned their attention to the tidying up process as they saw it of completing women's equality before the law.

The Feminist movement of the interwar years continued in practice to reflect the gap between women of the working class and bourgeois women. The popular image of womanhood was of emancipation achieved. The image of the Bright Young Thing (portrayed for example in the novels of Aldous Huxley and Evelyn Waugh) was complicated by falsely egalitarian images of woman imported from Hollywood; in the thirties, filmstars looked like the girl next door who was in her turn imitating the film stars.

That there had been real advance was undeniable. When the clothing trade tried to reintroduce long skirts after the war it failed dismally. Many women did make use of the new opportunities open to them. The Feminists did succeed in helping push through a number of legislative reforms in the interests of women. The Matrimonial Causes Act of 1923 made adultery by the man grounds for divorce; the Guardianship of Infants Act of 1925 equalized at last parental rights as between father and mother; the position of the wife seeking protection from her husband was also strengthened by the *Summary Jurisdiction (Separation and Maintenance) Act* of 1925. Other feminists worked in the Women's Institutes, hoping much from them as educational and democratic organizations.

The widening availability of birth control also suggested sexual emancipation, although the accounts of Marie Stopes and of Mary Stocks (1970) show that family planning was still looked on with horror among many sections of the population. The possibilities for the full sexual emancipation of women were further limited by the shortage of men and by the continuing belief in two sorts of women, the pure and the vicious. The

117

heroine of Machael Arlen's *The Green Hat* (1924), one of the best selling novels of the period, for example, could use men sexually but reserved her friendship and esteem for men who did not attract her; ultimately the conflict was too much and she ended it all by driving her Hispano-Suiza into a tree. Radclyffe Hall's notorious *The Well of Loneliness* (1927) portrayed lesbians as nothing but mutilated men.

Some progressive women, then as now, questioned the very validity of the feminist form of organization for the working women; Barbara Hutchins, for example wrote:

'The working woman, we should submit, has a far better chance to work out her economic salvation through solidarity and co-operation with her own class than by adopting the tactics and submitting to the tutelage of middle and upper class organisations which rise to no higher conception of women's work than that of ceaseless competition with men ...'   (Hutchins and Harrison 1926 : 198)

and she made a useful distinction between the position of middle-class women, which was one of exclusion and the situation of working-class women, which was one of exploitation. Winifred Holtby on the other hand, the most sensitive commentator of the period, understood the psychology of the slump and the contradiction between a consciousness of poverty and the existence of sexism, but remained clear that both must be fought, even in the difficult atmosphere of the thirties:

'Women who brought up their children on the assumption that the victory was secure ... now see the position once again challenged ... A sense of bitterness infects many public utterances, speeches and articles, made on the subject of women's position in the state. The economic slump has re-opened the question of women's right to earn. The political doctrine of the corporative State in Italy and Germany has inspired new pronouncements upon the function of the woman citizen. Psychological fashions arouse old controversies about the capacity of the female individual. The problems which feminists of the nineteenth century sought to solve along the lines of rationalism, individualism and democracy, present new difficulties in an age of mysticism, community and authority.' (Holtby 1934:7)

The inter-war period was characterized by repeated, halting attempts to cope with the unemployed and uninsured together with recurring efforts to impose cuts and economies. At the end of the war unemployment benefit schemes were still in their infancy. A group within the Ministry of Reconstruction had been appointed under Beveridge to plan for war-workers once the war was over, but their recommendation for a scheme of universal insurance was ignored (Gilbert 1970). Returning soldiers received an 'out-of-work donation' which in practice amounted to a paid up employment policy, and it soon seemed advisable in view of the general political unrest to extend the same scheme to civilian workers. When its first six month period expired, it was renewed for a further six months, and : ' "from the donation scheme dates the term 'dole' indiscriminately applied to the later insurance benefit also; and from it dates the conception of largesse to which all were entitled to share" ' (Gilbert 1970:60), wrote Beveridge in 1931.

A number of insurance and assistance measures were pushed through parliament, both during the period of industrial militancy up to the defeat of the General Strike in 1926, and afterwards (Hutt 1938). These culminated in the *1934 Unemployment Act* which reorganized the whole administration of unemployment monies on a national basis. The word 'pauper' had officially disappeared under an Act of 1931, and in practice the reality of the inter-war years was that the old Poor Law was continuously by-passed. But behind the halting story of legislation, cuts, and struggle was another and even more shameful one. The unemployed men of the Depression survived on the dole, eking out an apathetic existence, bought off, Bentley Gilbert suggests, by the Dole (which was after all fairly successful in containing the discontent of the working class, by comparison with other western European countries). But these men were the visible part of an iceberg; sunk below them were millions of toiling, downtrodden women, their lives the picture of the most dreadful neglect.

Despite the appearance of emancipation (confined in any case to the bourgeoisie), discrimination against women everywhere continued, and particularly in the two vital fields of employment and welfare. Yet the discrimination remained hidden, went unquestioned or, at most, seemed not to be accessible to parliamentary change. Throughout the social security system, for example, there was discrimination against women and especially against married women. Benefits for women were less than those for men, and women were treated as a bad health insurance risk. Because of pregnancy they were probably not an insurable group at all in the actuarial sense of the word; but the general confusion of the system – which was neither a proper insurance system nor a system of uncovenanted benefit – bore particularly harshly on women. In 1932 the *National Health Insurance and Contributory Pensions Act* actually reduced benefits for women, and at the same time the Approved Societies made an attempt to introduce another amendment whereby women, when they married, would have to requalify for health insurance as if they were new entrants by paying twenty-six weekly contributions, and being excluded from the maternity benefit for a year and from the disability benefit for two years. The women MPs, headed by Lady Astor, were able, with the support of the labour movement to campaign against this section of the Bill, which was in fact removed, but there was on the other hand no wider challenge to the general assumptions of the social security system in relation to women.

One of the intractable problems of the dole was that it often compared favourably to unskilled wage rates, particularly as the Assistance Board gave allowances for dependents. One way in which it seemed that it might be possible to deal with this was the Family Allowance, an idea which, borrowed from the Continent, appealed to two quite dissimilar groups in Britain. Of these, the first was a small group of progressive Tory MPs, led by Leo Amery (1953). For them, family allowances fitted in with still prevalent views on national efficiency and attempts to raise the birthrate, and in the thirties Amery used the widely publicized findings of John Boyd Orr, a nutritionist who claimed that twenty-five per cent of all children in Britain lacked *all* essential vitamins and minerals in their diet.

The second group was led by Eleanor Rathbone. She had worked for the COS before moving into the field of research into social problems. In 1913 she had published a report on *The*

Conditions of Widows under the Poor Law in Liverpool.
Widows at that time came under no scheme of national insurance whatsoever (this was rectified in 1925), and the position
of separated wives and cohabitees after the outbreak of war
further widened Eleanor Rathbone's perspective on the problem
of the mother bringing up her children alone. She began to
evolve the theory of motherhood as a service to the community,
and believed that 'society should substitute a system of more
direct payment of the costs of its own renewal'. She herself
linked her ideas of Family Allowances, which she called the
Endowment of Motherhood, firmly with the problem of equal
pay. She believed that women should have equal pay with men
and her answer to the argument that men need a larger wage
because it must be a 'family wage' was to equalize the situation
of the wage earner with a family and the wage earner with no
dependants by means of family endowment, an allowance for
each child. In 1917 she established a small committee consisting
of feminists and Labour Party members, the Family Endowment
Committee, to put out a statement of the argument for the
family allowance. This pamphlet, *Equal Pay and the Family*,
appeared in 1918. The Committee was then enlarged into the
Family Endowment Society, with more supporters, of whom
Beveridge (at that time Director of the London School of
Economics), was one. After the war she became President of
the National Union of Women's Suffrage Societies, which now
became the National Union of Societies for Equal Citizenship.
This change in name reflected a significant debate amongst
feminists between those who wanted to continue to work
solely for women's equality and those who felt that, this objective having been achieved, they should now be free to devote
their energies to the other political and philanthropic causes
dear to their hearts. There was further debate and considerable
disagreement over Family Endowment, but this was eventually
adopted as policy. Eleanor Rathbone's arguments in favour of
the scheme never lost a wider perspective on feminism. She did
not wish to see motherhood as an inseparable part of continued
marital dependency for women. She realized that in order for
women to have true equality, their demands had to go beyond
mere emancipation and equality before the law (Stocks 1949).
Yet the whole nature of family allowances and the endowment

of motherhood is ambivalent, and it is not surprising that it met with opposition from, on the one hand, bourgeois feminists such as Dame Millicent Fawcett, who feared that such a step would undermine family responsibility, and Ellen Wilkinson (Amery 1953) the left-wing Labour MP on the other, who saw family allowances as an attack on wages (see Stocks (1949) for a different account of Wilkinson's position).

John Boyd Orr was not alone in his knowledge of undernourishment and consequent sickness amongst working-class families, particularly the unemployed. Wal Hannington quotes at length from the reports of Medical Officers of Health across the country to prove its extent, but he, unlike many other writers on the subject understood its meaning in terms of working-class life, and attacked not Boyd Orr but others for discussing working-class diets in the pseudo-scientific way which was in fact a form of censure of working-class women, and highly ideological:

'We frequently come up against insidious propaganda, which I believe has been encouraged by the Ministry of Health, to the effect that it is not the amount of income to the household that is too low, but ... the ignorance of the average working-class housewife in regard to food values and the art of cooking, resulting in the loss of the nutritive qualities of the food, which is responsible for the present ill-health that pervades so many working-class homes. It is indeed interesting to read of the well-to-do woman assuming the right to instruct the working-class mother on the way she shall spend the 4s. or less on twenty-one meals a week ...

When the average housewife goes out to spend her very limited means on food, she does not work out whether this or that food contains this or that amount of calories or vitamins. She has a general knowledge of what is nutritious, but at the same time she has to plan her expenditure in such a way that if possible she can put food on the table for her family which satisfies their hunger – even if it may not contain the same amount of calories as a smaller and less satisfying amount of food ... The sacrifice of the mother for the child is quite a common thing amongst working-class families. When there is not enough food in the home to satisfy all, the mother will go without in order to allow her child to have more. In 1934 a sanatorium superintendent stated to a Press correspondent, when asked for his impressions about the type of patients being admitted to the sanatorium: "Among the adults there has been an increase in the number of young people admitted, especially women, suffering from an acute type of tuberculosis. They appear to have no immunity, and their resistance seemed to be completely overcome".'   (Hannington 1963:60–2)

On the whole, however, public concern centred rather on children than on mothers. The search for a 'scientific' approach to child care was in evidence and there was a continued extension of provisions for mothers and babies and for children. In 1918 the *Maternity and Child Welfare Act* established local authority services for expectant and nursing mothers, and for children under five years of age. The *Midwives Act* of 1902 had laid down standards for training, maintained a register, and prevented the untrained from practising, but midwives had remained private practitioners. Already by 1918 there were three thousand health visitors working for the local authorities, and the *Midwives Act* of 1936 made it obligatory for local authorities to ensure that there was an adequate number of midwives in their areas. But the 1918 Act was never fully implemented; Sylvia Pankhurst wrote that by 1927 only 57 local authorities were supplying home helps during confinements, and she was critical of public attitudes towards the service, which she felt 'should be raised to the dignity of a profession' (1930). Sylvia Pankhurst was also aware of the way in which the ambivalences and conflict of the period were mirrored in the care of mothers, babies, and children. Anxiety over the declining birthrate and over the high, and for some years rising, mortality rate for women after birth, was at war with other concerns, not all economic:

'The Maternity and Child Welfare Act of 1918, if it were fully applied, could aid substantially in reducing to the general level the excessive mortality amongst the children of ... forlorn young [unmarried] mothers; but the fear of "encouraging" their condition militates against applying the provisions of the Act to those whose need is greatest.'

(Pankhurst 1930:120)

(Yet even in the thirties it seems (Oakley 1975) women still preferred the services of the 'handywoman' – untrained female midwives – to those of GP, hospital, and even state-certified midwife.)

Perhaps the most striking testimony to the exploitation of these women is Margery Spring Rice's *Working Class Wives* (1939), the Report of the Women's Health Enquiry Committee. Filled with examples of the squalor and undernourishment endemic to their lives, together with the dreadful housing conditions and chronic ill-health, often related to multiple pregnancies, it comments on a general passive acceptance of these conditions as inevitable. Even more pathetic are the complaints of monotony, dreariness, and depression as the women grew older and their burden of work slackened without being replaced by any new interests. Yet the Report also commented on the way in which working-class women appeared to cling to some of the worst aspects of their situation:

'Examples of this are provided in the great difficulty which occurs in persuading women to go into hospital for their confinements; although trained home helps can be provided to look after the father and children the mothers show an inherent disinclination to entrust their homes even temporarily to the care of someone else. Again mothers themselves have often been the first to oppose the granting of school meals for their children, holding that it is unnatural for the children to eat away from home and that they prefer to prepare the food themselves. Another example is the opposition from many parents with which the Ministry of Labour was met in the initial stages of their scheme to remove adolescent wage earners from the distressed areas. The boys and girls after leaving school are placed in hostels in different parts of the country with the object of training them for and placing them in jobs which could be found for them more easily in these districts. The Ministry has had to devote much time and propaganda to breaking down the parental prejudice against this "unnatural" disintegration of the family.'

(Spring Rice 1939:14 n.)

The training hostels for young unemployed workers provide a good example of the contradictory attitude of the State towards the family. All modern British administrations have made conscious efforts to preserve the family; yet at times of crisis it may have to be destroyed in the interests of the preservation of capitalism. And the mocking and patronizing tone of the extract quoted above goes a long way to explain why the recipients have so often rejected State welfarism; it comes in an authoritarian form, seeming to show up the inadequacies in particular of the woman, of her housekeeping and mothering capacities, even introducing a rival into her house. It is utilitarian and lacks all real respect, despite its mouthings about the sanctity of the family, for personal affection, as it lacks all understanding of the bitter reality of working-class lives.

SEVEN

Welfare & war

Twice in this century world war on a scale not hitherto experienced has necessitated a mobilization of our whole society in a way that is also new. There has been a good deal of debate amongst historians as to the long-term effects of this on society; some, amongst them Richard Titmuss (1950; also Marwick 1973), have attributed important developments in welfare provision to the influence of total war, others have sought to demonstrate its unimportance as an accelerator of social change (Milward (1971) discusses this debate); I shall seek in this chapter to show the way in which war has revealed quite glaringly the contradictory nature of women's lives, has shown new possibilities for social organization, yet has also revealed why these possibilities are cast aside once peace has returned. In general, total war, and particularly the Second World War, appears as a period of excitement, an upsurge of energy, participation, and co-operative effort (Longmate 1973). Arthur Marwick (1968) likens war to a wedding – a heightened experience offsetting by contrast the dull routine of everyday life, startling and rebellious. For women it has been like marriage in a different sense, since for them it has reinforced the conventions while purporting to offer new freedoms.

During both World Wars in Britain the transformation of women's lives was simply one aspect of the complete transformation of social life and also of the economy. In both wars state rationalization and control of the economy was necessary. By 1918 ninety per cent of total imports, the home production of food, coal, and most other raw materials was controlled by the government. It controlled food distribution by means of rationing, and allocated raw materials. In the summer of 1916 the Federation of British Industries was formed, and the appreciation by businessmen of the advantages of state control was reflected in its support of collectivization – indeed, wartime state control had nothing to do with socialism, but was rather an amalgam of business and the state. As the *Glasgow Herald* put it, 'the conduct of the modern war is simply a form of business', and should therefore be run by businessmen, while according to Beveridge, the Ministry of Munitions created in 1915 by Lloyd George was:

> ' "from first to last a businessman's organisation, [intended] to liberate the munitions industries from military direction, and the restrictions of established official routine, and to hand over the task of guiding and co-ordinating these developments to prominent businessmen familiar with industrial problems." '
>
> (Hinton 1973:29)

Manpower and the control of the labour force was the most acute problem of all, and it was here that state control utilized some of the welfare apparatus set up by the Liberals:

> ' "The Act of 1909 had anticipated the War ... (together with the Insurance Act it ensured that) the numbers, classes, and even the distribution of the workers were known with accuracy. Moreover the Exchanges had acquired a special and intimate acquaintance with the labour engaged in these trades

and had formed, in many cases, close association with the employers." '   (Hinton 1973:30)

Furthermore the civil servants who had in peace time organized social insurance were now placed in charge of the organization of labour control, with William Beveridge in charge.

In the Second World War as in the First the productivity of British industry and agriculture accelerated, although at the long-term cost of the replacement and upkeep of capital equipment, and there were again scientific and technological advances and new methods of mass-production, of industrial control and management, and of design and quality control. There was more thorough-going control of the consumer end of the economy than had occurred in the First World War, with rent control and food subsidies introduced to counteract inflation, together with stringent rationing to ensure fair shares of scarce goods in the community. This was indeed a form of welfarism in that it was a social benefit which in its turn had a reward for the State in the shape of social peace. Although it was not the only or the most important reason, it was one factor contributing towards the social peace that had been absent in the First World War, but which was a notable feature of the Second.

More important in this respect was the role of Ernest Bevin (Bullock 1967), appointed Minister of Labour by Winston Churchill. In peacetime a trades union boss on the right wing of the Labour Party, Bevin was able to act as conciliator between government and unions. His appointment and the way in which he carried out his work also pointed the way forward for the future organization of British capital, marking as it did a further step in organized consultation between government and unions. A tripartite system of government, employers, and labour in joint consultation became the desired method of managing industrial friction and economic problems. In the long-run this was a move in the direction of the further incorporation of the union hierarchy into government and away from the function of the trades union as an organization to defend the worker against his employer; it made for social peace in the short-run partly because Bevin's strategy was to rely on what he called 'voluntaryism' and to avoid any form of industrial conscription, in which even Beveridge, a wholehearted believer in compulsion, was forced to agree with him: 'Unreasoning rejection of industrial discipline even in war, however dangerous in itself, is perhaps the last ditch against totalitarian rule for all time, in war and peace thereafter' (Beveridge 1953:162). Bevin also insisted that there must be no wage freeze, and that collective bargaining must remain the means by which wages were settled. By the time the manpower shortage in 1941 had made further measures necessary, Bevin's approach had secured the co-operation of the population and thus made possible the new measures of the *National Service (No. 2) Act*, which included the conscription of women into the Auxiliary Forces, and the obligation of all men and women between the ages of eighteen and sixty to do some sort of war work.

Much of the labour unrest in the First World War had centred round the issue of dilution, the replacement of skilled workers by semi-skilled or unskilled workers. The process was not simply the result of war, but was a process that had been gradually revolutionizing industry since the 1880s. The old craft workers were being slowly ousted by new techniques; the war was however an opportunity in the eyes of some industrialists to strengthen their hand against the unions. In practice, dilution most often meant the introduction of female labour into the factories, so there was a struggle of men against women too (Hinton 1973). The threat was a real one, and cannot be dismissed purely as paranoia on the part of the male workers due to their sexism and prejudice. Some men, moreover, did understand the importance for women of work; John Maclean (Milton 1973), for example, understood the importance of unionizing them as the only means of preventing them from being used as scab labour. On the other hand the National Federation of Women Workers agreed to withdraw its members at the end of the war from those occupations claimed by the Association of Skilled Engineers in return for the latter's offer to act jointly with them in wage negotiations during the war; opposition to women workers remained strong in the unions and women's labour organizations were in fact excluded from some of the negotiations surrounding dilution (Andrews and Hobbs 1918). The compromise reached was in fact that dilution should be for the duration of the War only. 1,659,000 women were added to the workforce between April 1915 and July 1918. According to official statistics 1,816,000 women were taking men's places by 1918. During the first year of the war they replaced men mostly in transport, the retail trade and clerical work. Then as more and more men left for the Front, they increasingly entered all spheres of employment, and in spite of dilution agreements it seems that there was a permanent acceleration of the trend towards the employment of women. For instance, in 1911 703,000 women were employed in the clothing trade, and in 1921 only 503,000, but this reflected a decrease in sweated female labour in the garment trade and the total number of women in gainful employment increased by 234,000 during the same period. In the shipbuilding industry 8,000 women were employed in 1911 and 42,000 in 1921. In the civil service the number rose even more strikingly, from 33,000 to 102,000. The greatest gain was in transport, where the number of women employees increased from 18,000 in 1914 to 177,000 in 1918. Many of these women had previously been in domestic service, which lost 400,000 during the war. (Yet domestic service was far from wiped out by the First War, and in 1931 36 per cent of the female working force was still engaged in domestic labour.)

At first it was believed that women were not as efficient as men except on routine and repetitive work, but as they became more experienced employers began to think highly of their work. The Report of the Chief Inspector of Factories and Workshops for 1916 commented on some of the effects of substitution in the words of the Principal Lady Inspector, Miss Anderson, who wrote:

' "It appears that the one absolute limit in the replacement of men by women lies in those heavy occupations and processes where adaptation of plant or appliances cannot be effected so as to bring them within the compass even of selected women, of physical capacity above the normal. Very surprising, however, is the outcome of careful selection, even in fairly heavy work ... 'If they will stick this they will stick anything,' a manager is reported as saying of the grit and pluck of the women in a gas works in the recent severe weather ... It is permissible to wonder whether some of the surprise and admiration freely expressed in many quarters over new proofs of women's physical capacity and endurance is not in part attributable to lack of knowledge or appreciation of the very heavy and strenuous nature of much of normal pre-war work for women, domestic and industrial." '

(Andrews and Hobbs 1918:40)

The freely expressed admiration did not result in equal pay. The Government appeared, although rather reluctantly, to support the principle of equal pay for equal work, but women never reached parity with men and instead the determining factor was what it was believed the industry would be able to support after the War.

During the Second World War the exodus of women from their homes to the factories did not prove so contentious, although Britain took the conscription of women to greater lengths than any other country, the Soviet Union and Nazi Germany not excluded. This was partly because of the sense of 'national unity' which over-rode class struggle, and partly because Bevin's work simply accelerated the existing trend for more women to work outside the home. Before the First World War there had been nearly 5½ million women in employment and during that war the figure had risen to 7½ million. This number fell off immediately after the war, but the rise was resumed and continued throughout the depression. It would have led to about 6¾ million women being employed in 1943 had there been no war. In fact the official estimate of the number of women in employment in that year was again 7½ million, so the trend was only hastened to the extent of about ¾ million women (Calder 1971). The women were noticeable, however, because they were not just in paid employment, but were once again entering the preserve of men:

'Between June 1939 and December 1943 the number of women in engineering and allied industries had risen from 411,000 to over 1,500,000, from 18 per cent to 30 per cent of the total labour force, and four out of five of these were on semi-skilled or skilled work.'

(Bullock 1967:63)

Bevin recognized that women's pay would have to improve, but equal pay was never achieved any more than it had been in the First War. Where an equal pay agreement had been reached, as in the engineering industries it was usually evaded or circumvented. In January 1944 women in metal work and engineering earned an average £3/10/0 as compared with a man's wage of over £5. The railway companies refused to pay women the rate for the job on the grounds that they had been unable to find any other industry in which this principle was applied (Calder 1971).

It does appear, too, that women were seen as shouldering this burden for the duration of the war only, and also still as adjuncts of their fighting men-folk:

'[Bevin] made a special appeal to the women to join the auxiliary forces and to take on jobs in industry. "I saw one headline the other day," he remarked at Leicester, "which said: Bevin wants 100,000 women, the State to keep the children." If they had husbands or sweethearts in the Forces they could help to make the weapons to equip them; this was the quickest way to end the war and get their menfolk home again.'   (Calder 1971:76)

Similarly a war-work recruitment poster headed 'London shop-girl Attacks Nazis' continued:

'With the shop half-empty and so little to sell, my old job began to seem pointless and useless. My boy is in the RAF – so they arranged at the Employment Exchange for me to train for War Work. Soon I was passed to a factory for a worthwhile job helping to make big bombers – those that go to Berlin. And Jim has just got his wings. Who knows? I might have worked on the plane he flies . . .'
                                                (Longmate 1973)

The departure of men to the front and the exodus of women into the factories focused public attention on conditions in the factories and on conditions of home life alike. Both wars revealed deficiencies in factory welfare; in the First War particularly, the presence of 'ladies' made conditions such as the absence of proper washing facilities, lavatories, and rest rooms no longer tolerable. It was found, too, that better conditions in the factories made for increased output as well as greater contentment among the workers. The welfare officers who were appointed were however, unpopular. Mary Macarthur as Secretary of the National Federation of Women Workers described 'welfare' as 'the most unpopular word in the terminology of the factory worker' and pointed to the aspects of social control and manipulation implicit in the work:

' "The good welfare worker was the most dangerous because she was most likely to be successful in reducing independence and in turning the workers from trades unionism; she was a more efficient kind of slave driver ... While some women supervisors in the future – like some forewomen in the past – will do much to safeguard and improve our girls' working lives, others will begin their career full of queer notions as to discipline and open-work stockings and firmly persuaded ... that trades unionism is of the devil." '

(Andrews and Hobbs 1918:159)

As a result of the war experience, welfare work was established and became another offshoot of social work, a number of courses for welfare supervisors being started at some of the newer universities. Similarly, in the Second World War there was the same story of better conditions in the factories leading to higher productivity, and factory welfare remained important after the war when full employment and labour shortages made welfare considerations a necessity, particularly in the climate of the Welfare State. Also, in the Second War especially, it was recognized that welfare needed to go beyond the factory if women were to be brought out of their homes. One reason for this was the decline in family size:

'Of the women between 45 and 54 who were married at the ages of 20 to 24 and had been married for 25–30 years in 1911, 71 per cent had four or more children, and 41 per cent had seven or more; only about 5 per cent had no children.

Of the married women who in 1951 were roughly the same age and who had been married at the same ages for roughly the same length of time, only about 25 per cent had four or more children and only 5 per cent seven or more; nearly 11 per cent had no children. It is true that far more children born to the earlier generation died in childhood, but it nonetheless remains true that the family circle of 1910 or thereabouts was very much wider than it was thirty or forty years later.'

(Ferguson and Fitzgerald 1949:1)

This meant a corresponding decline in self-help and mutual help, which, although masked in peacetime by working-class neighbourliness (and in middle-class families by the existence of servants, of whom there were still more than 1½ million in 1939) became evident in wartime with the dispersal of families and the need for all members of the family to go out to work. Mobilization was so total that only the very young, the very old, and the chronically sick or disabled were left without work in the community, the very ones of course who needed other people to look after them.

The care of children in all its forms was a major feature of all the wartime welfare schemes. Married women with children under fourteen living at home were never compelled to work, but both for economic reasons (for instance the allowances to the familes of servicemen remained pitiably small throughout the war) and for patriotic reasons many of these women worked at least part-time; about 2,160,000 extra women aged between 14 and 59 had entered the workforce by 1943; this figure counts two part-time workers as one, so the number of individual women going out to work for at least part of the day would have been nearer to three million. In addition many women over sixty were working and around one million women were working as unpaid volunteers in canteens, nurseries, the WVS and other organizations.

Day nurseries therefore became essential. Although the Treasury was at first unenthusiastic because it was feared that the many supporters of the nursery 'movement' might use the scheme as leverage to push for far more comprehensive provision in the future than would normally have been approved, twelve-hour nurseries were eventually provided, and this was done under the control of central government. Those most hostile to nurseries argued more on economic and moralistic grounds than on the grounds of the damage to the child's emotional growth, asserting that nurseries did not actually release an economically justifiable number of women for the factories and that it would have been better and simpler to send the nursery workers into war-work directly. But these were often the older and less geographically mobile women workers, so that this argument did not necessarily hold. In any case it was equally possible to argue that the provision of nurseries was in part an expression of the right of mothers to contribute to the war effort, and an acknowledgement of the responsibilities of the State in wartime.

Day nurseries, canteens, better maternity services which evolved out of some of the evacuation schemes, and the provision of special rations for pregnant women, nursing mothers, and babies all related to the necessity for an expanded and healthy labour force in wartime and for a new generation of healthy babies to replace the loss of life inevitable in war. Revelations as to the nature and deficiencies of working-class home life were also a feature of both wars. Sylvia Pankhurst, for example, unlike many of the Suffragettes, continued her political and welfare work in the East End during the First War, as well as campaigning against the war itself. In particular she was active in securing proper allowances for the dependants of the men who had gone to fight, and in this struggle, which also involved agitating against the delays of the Poor Law Guardians, and practices such as police spying on soldiers' wives and families to see if they were 'worthy' of their allowances, she came across so many starved and sickly mothers and children that she opened four mother-and-baby clinics, also a cost-price restaurant where the destitute could eat free. She and her helpers were also drawn into various forms of advocacy in trying to sort out delays and difficulties over pensions and allowances, although she always where possible, encouraged the women to represent themselves and to accompany her on deputations to Cabinet ministers and government bodies, and, when there, to speak for themselves of their own oppression. Later on, more general public concern was expressed about the home life of women and children during the war, juveniles giving rise to special anxiety. It was felt that the long hours being worked by women, and the absence of fathers – indeed effectively of both parents – must be having a bad effect on both older and younger children. The home, it was feared, was being undermind. Yet while this might have been the case:

'even the traditional responsibility placed on many women by the absence of their men folk seems to have been one of the stimulating influences which are said to have "transformed" the personality of the average factory women. As a class, they have grown more confident, more independent, more interested in impersonal issues.'

(Andrews and Hobbs 1918:9)

Their children might be running wild, might be illegally employed under-age, might be taking to crime and evading school, but women were experiencing a new freedom. Since the 'deterioration of character' amongst juveniles was specifically linked with the new conditions in the home, it was to be expected that once the war was over women would be encouraged to return to their traditional sphere, which happened; in the meantime, the freedom of women posed itself in the form of a direct conflict between their own interests and those of their families.

During the Second World War it was evacuation (Titmuss 1950; Calder 1971) that, in the words of one report, 'flooded the dark places with light' (Hygiene Committee of the Women's Group on Public Welfare 1942). The first confrontation of the war was not that of the British with the Nazis, but of the politer parts of England with the slums; a class confrontation. As might have been expected, the parents who took advantage of the Government's 'public' evacuation scheme tended to be the poorer members of the community, for the better off, and those who had relations in other parts of the country to whom they could turn in many cases preferred to do so. The result was hosts who were often not only horrified but also angered by the behaviour and appearance of the children they were being asked to care for. There were children who did not know how to use a knife and fork, children who had never slept in a bed and were too frightened to do so, and children who not only were not provided with nightclothes, but were sewn into their underwear (Calder 1971). Worse still were slum mothers who smoked, went to the pub, and used obscene language. The well-bred inhabitants of quiet provincial and rural communities took refuge in moral censure as the only way of coping with the stench of the slums that was being thrust beneath their noses. Remote and alien to them was the reality of life in those slums, where mothers could neither afford fresh vegetables nor cook them in a tenement with shared cooker and one cold tap three flights down. They did not believe that unemployed families could never afford proper shoes for their children, nor understand that rough manners were the natural outcome of the public, brutal life where all could hear the quarrels, love-making, and painful illnesses of their neighbours. There were additional immediate fac   king the first meeting between town and country hos   d at the end of a very long, hot day in tr   rs, lavatories, or water, to be met by   all rescuing the victims of an ac   ally been dropped. The ro   etic refugees from a war-   ngry reality of messy chil-   o class antagonisms were   among children, as Jonathan Mi   emembers :

'Th   like   hose horrible figures in M. R. Jan   called   earts – grieving little phantoms with   r their hearts. There were at least two   st hearts in each of the towns or vil-lages   can still remember their shrunken Fair Isle j   down from one of the children of the famil   ey were staying. And they always seemed to hav   cuee colds, as well, with a thick jade drib-ble co   ne nostril. They were also much stronger and mu   ggressive than we were; despite their pallor and wea   their grief. Possibly because of it. To com-fortable   class children like myself these displaced in-fants were   er like werewolves. That is to say they were strong *because* of their weakness and dangerous *because* they were sick. They also represented a living embodiment of the condition which nannies threaten one with. They were, after all, the protagonists of banishment, so that look-ing at them in all their lost wolfishness, one could see an image of oneself, turned out of the house and sent away for naughtiness.'   (Johnson 1968 : 203)

The psychological effect on children of evacuation was to have important repercussions on later social policy, but at the time it seems not to have occurred either to hosts or planners that some of the problems, particularly bed-wetting, might have been due to the emotional effects of the separation of small children from their parents. In this context, Bowlby, writing on the psychological and emotional implications of evacuation for the Fabian Society (Padley and Cole 1940) could appear as progressive, since the planners, as Margaret Cole points out in the same survey had not even acknowledged the existence of psychology:

'Psychologically the scheme failed to appeal, partly, I suggest because it was drawn up by minds that were military, male and middle-class ... Surely only male calculations could have so confidently assumed that working-class wives would be content to leave their husbands indefinitely to look after themselves, and only middle-class parents, accustomed to shoo their children out of sight and reach at the earliest possible opportunity could have been so astonished to find that working-class parents were violently unwilling to part with with theirs.'   (Padley and Cole 1940:4)

The full implications of Bowlby's approach was not yet evident, especially at the time when enuresis, headlice, and inadequate clothing often met with anger and contempt. One contemporary survey, while making the point that the complaints about evacuees related to only a small proportion and to individuals from all parts of the country, and while acknowledging the real poverty of the 'submerged tenth' now revealed, displays especially bleakly the typical reaction of class prejudice and moral condemnation in tones reminiscent of the COS:

'Evacuation was to ... bring home to the national consciousness that the "submerged tenth" described by Charles Booth still exists in our towns like a hidden sore, poor, dirty and crude in its habits, an intolerable and degrading burden to decent people forced by poverty to neighbour with it.

Within this group are the "problem families", always on the edge of pauperism and crime, riddled with mental and physical defects, in and out of the Courts for child neglect, a menace to the community ... Next to the problem families come those which may be described as grey rather than black; they are dirty and unwholesome in their habits through lack of personal discipline and social standard, often combined in the past or present with poverty and discouraging environment. Most of them are capable of improvement in better circumstances and if educated in a wide sense ... It was said that the mothers were dirty, verminous, idle and extravagant; that they could not hold a needle and did not know the rudiments of cooking and housecraft, and that they had no control over their young children, who were untrained and animal in their habits. Some of these women were said to be foulmouthed, bullying and abusive, given to drinking and frequenting public houses, insanitary in their habits and loose in their morals.'

(Hygiene Committee of the Women's Group on
Public Welfare 1942)

and, significantly, wasteful spending was considered to be the result of a lack of the 'heroism with which the vast majority of the working class are said to have faced the hard days of unemployment'.

Richard Titmuss (1950) has pointed out and described in detail how many of the welfare provisions set up around or as a result of evacuation (and the homelessness caused by bombing to a lesser extent) tended to develop into social welfare provision. Residential nurseries were one example of this, for while the problem of broken homes was not new, it had not been an officially recognized area of specialized State intervention before the war, and the *Poor Law* had been the only State resource for children in need of full-time care. Even had a particular scandal over a foster child who died of neglect not precipitated the setting up of the Curtis Committee after the war, the nature of State provision for children whose parents for one reason or another could not care for them was bound to have become a focus for concern in the post-war climate of opinion when the rebuilding of family life was stressed, and in the light of the deficiencies revealed by the wartime experience. Nurseries in general ceased to be an emergency evacuation provision, and whereas in 1940, 47 per cent of applications for admission were as the result of air raids and only 21 and 15 per cent because of parents in hospital or a mother wishing to work, by 1943 the proportions had changed with no children entering nurseries because of air raids, but 39 per cent because of parental illness and 43 per cent because the mother wanted to work.

The success of trained social workers during the war in

organizing emergency services for children and those who had been bombed out, especially the latter, established them in the eyes of the State as a specialized skilled group, when the disarray of war threw up personal problems requiring special attention. (For instance, one unexpected problem was that of the many old people found to be shelter-bound, bombed out, or simply too frightened to emerge, often decrepit, with nothing of their own and no-one to care for them.) Richard Titmuss sees in their work a 'new concept of the relationship between public agencies and the public served', and feels that their work during the War paved the way for their enhanced influence after it.

So the upheaval of the War and the excessive mobility of the population revealed many gaps and inadequacies in social welfare provision together with depths of poverty and degradation those in power had hitherto been able to ignore, and aroused much interest in, particularly, the care of children and the old. Better pay and full employment also brought renewed hope and optimism and a new spirit of radicalism was fostered by the War. Soldiers especially were receptive to talk of change. 'Progressive' capitalists recognized the potential dangers of this and the likely necessity of future concessions (Calder 1971), and post-war reconstruction became again, as it had been during the First World War, a focus for discussion and of the hopes of all.

The two key discussion documents on post-war reconstruction were the *Beveridge Report* (1942) followed two years later by the *White Paper on Employment Policy*. The *Beveridge Report* was a best-seller when it was first published. Greeted as a wonderful, transforming, and revolutionary document, with its promise of a minimum income, however meagre, to all as of right, it gave the population something positive to fight for apart from simply the defeat of Hitler; it seemed to promise a rosy future and was greeted with what one more cynical commentator described as 'a deluge of slush'. Yet this may not have represented the real feelings of many ordinary people. At least one study of wartime opinion found that working-class attitudes to family allowances, which formed an adjunct to Beveridge's proposals, were far from enthusiastic. This study (Slater and Woodside 1951), although not published until 1951, was based on a survey of working-class soldiers and their wives during the war. The authors make no claim that their sample is representative, but it was a fairly large one. These authors found that on the question of government propaganda to persuade couples to have more babies both the men and their wives showed 'the strongest resentment':

> 'They showed indignation that the production of large numbers of children could be expected of them as a duty. "I want some fun out of life; I'm not interested in raising the birthrate" says a wife of 22 with one child. Almost all thought of (family allowances) as an effort to boost the birthrate, rather than as an amelioration of hardship for the more prolific. They were taken as an inducement, a bribe, a payment – and a very inadequate one: "the wife said *she* wasn't going to have a baby for five bob a week", "I'd like to see *them* keep a baby on five shillings". No-one thought that the allowances would have any effect in encouraging fertility generally, or that they would influence their own decision. They were judged in relation to their income and standards, and the real cost of a child. Many women, and some men too, stressed the need for day nurseries, and not only as a wartime measure. This can be seen as an aspect of the general tendency to demand a lessening of the drudgery connected with rearing a family.' (Slater and Woodside 1951:189)

On the other hand, the writers noted that the men did not welcome the increased independence of their wives which had been brought about by the war. One reason, no doubt, for the warm welcome given the Beveridge Report was that it located the woman firmly within the home. Popular propaganda echoed this, and, looking ahead, resorted to the old remedy of education for motherhood:

> ' "Wives", says Dr Summerskill, "are still treated officially as unpaid domestic helps ... their share in the running of a home is in fact as important as the husband's; yet, financially they are entirely dependent, and in many households they have to ask for money as a favour.
>
> We must emancipate women inside the home as well as outside it ... for this decline in families is a great Women's Revolt. We must give the non-earning wife a legal right to a

share of her husband's income, and so a real status in her own home. Then, family life will have prestige again ... Probably the most constructive thing we could do now is through education – we could encourage people to think about family life at a much younger age than they do at present. There are very few schools in Britain where any sort of domesticity is taught at all. At the best girls' schools where academic teaching may be very high indeed, there is often no cooking, dressmaking or domestic science – let alone mothercraft – in the curriculum. It seems lopsided that many girls should read Greek and Latin but have no notion how to fry an egg. If a bigger proportion of school time were given over to teaching the home-making subjects, wouldn't girls – and boys too – grow up with a wish to use their knowledge in making a real family life?" '

(Hopkinson 1972: 146–48)

wrote Anne Scott James hopefully in *Picture Post*. But in the Slater and Woodside survey large families were associated with drudgery and poverty, and a knowledge of contraception was widespread. Women at least were enjoying their new freedom, and were more interested in life outside the home than in housecraft lessons.

The *Beveridge Report* was based on a Keynesian approach to the economy. Throughout the depression Keynes had argued that full employment was possible provided there was State intervention either in the shape of public investments (e.g. in schools, hospitals, or roads) or in the shape of a subsidy for mass consumption (e.g. introduction of family allowances, reduction in indirect taxes) or both. This was to be paid by borrowing rather than taxation which would have adversely affected both private investment and consumption. In 1940 Keynes wrote *How to Pay for the War*, he was brought into the Treasury in the summer of that year, and in 1941 the Chancellor of the Exchequer presented the first Keynesian budget. What Keynes now proposed was the same strategy as that appropriate for dealing with slump, but in reverse, to curb inflation; in order to hold back consumer spending he advocated greatly increased taxes, which would also finance part of the war effort. Some of these taxes would be repaid after the war by means of post-war credits. The 1944 *White Paper on Employment Policy* made proposals for the future, and envisaged in a rather simplistic fashion that after the war the trade cycle would continue, but would be modified by government action to compensate for the down-turn by timing its own investment to coincide with periods when private investment slackened. Also published in 1944 was the *TUC Interim Report on Post War Reconstruction*; the 1944 *White Paper* was accepted by both major political parties as well as by both sides of industry all of whom had come by the end of the War to accept a measure of planning (Rogow 1955; PEP 1952). It is also important to remember that the *Beveridge Report* was by no means simply a response on the part of the ruling class to possible future unrest; on the contrary it was a response to demands from the labour movement:

'The General Council of the TUC had for some time been pressing the Government for a comprehensive review of social insurance. A deputation of the Council received in February 1941 ... had stressed particularly the inadequacy of health insurance cash benefit as compared with other benefits, and its inequalities from one contributor to another under the Approved Society system. They criticised also the provision for medical treatment, both by general practitioners and in the hospitals. They pointed out that their hope of getting incidental examination of health insurance through the Royal Commission on Workmen's Compensation appointed in 1938 was being defeated; the employers had said that during the war they were too busy to give evidence and in the middle of 1940 the Commission had suspended its work. The TUC deputation of February 1941 were concerned primarily with health insurance, but they stressed the wider aspects of the problem as it presented itself to the ordinary man: "From the insured person's point of view the problem is how to provide an income when he loses his wages, and at present that central fact is dealt with by a whole lot of schemes purporting to deal with the same problem, but each providing a different kind of remedy." '

(Beveridge 1953:296)

The TUC demand was therefore a modest one, the rationalization and improvement of the existing insurance system.

How was it then that the implementation of this modest demand, along with the full employment policies that also seemed to all sides to be a necessary part of the post-war settlement, came to be elevated into a special form of post-capitalist or even socialist society, the Welfare State? What were the forces that led to the creation of a powerful ideology of welfare in post-war Britain?

> 'No socialist who saw it will forget the blissful dawn of July 1945. The great war in Europe had ended; the lesser war in Asia might be ending soon. This background to the scene in Britain naturally deepened the sense of release and breath-taking opportunity. And those who had served the British Labour movement for generations, renewing their faith after each disaster, in 1919, in 1926 and 1931, had their own special cause for exultation. When the scale of the Labour Party's victory became known on the night of 26th July, bonfires were lit, people danced in the streets, and young and old crowded into halls all over the country to acclaim their elected Standard bearers ... Varying elements and expectations combined to make the Labour Party, but one theme united them as never before. Eyes were fixed on the promise of a new society. Suddenly the vision of the Socialist pioneers had been given substance and historic impetus by the radical political ferment of wartime.'   (Foot 1963 : 17)

'We've won the war – now let's win the Peace' shouted the Labour Party posters pasted across the bomb sites. Another electioneering cartoon made the point more elaborately, with its drawing of a demobbed soldier and his young wife banging on the counter of the Tory Peace Stores. Under the counter are hidden 'jobs', 'proper medical attention', 'good homes', 'decent schools' – all 'the fruits of victory', marked 'reserved for the rich and privileged'. Soldier: 'What d'you mean, you're out of stock? I've paid for these twice – once in 1914 and once in 1939' (Sissons & French 1963).

On the one hand then, was the overwhelming Labour victory at the polls, which was a genuine mandate for change and represented a radical spirit in the population. There was also the desire of the Labour Party leaders to believe, and have it generally believed, that their government was socialist. On the other side was the ruling class, perhaps not too disturbed, once it had got over the shock or rejection by 'the mob' (as Churchill put it), that its opponents had what was bound to be the thankless task of clearing up the mess after the war. The Right was as anxious as the Labour Party that the Attlee government should be seen – in the most negative sense – as the party of Socialism, equated with petty tyranny, controls, and planners' blight. The Press waged an unceasing Red Labour propaganda campaign throughout the years Labour was in power (Rogow 1955), and was supplemented by organizations such as Aims of Industry (responsible for Tate and Lyle's massive anti-nationalization campaign). Not only popular literature, such as the novels of Angela Thirkell (*Love Among the Ruins* (1948) is one of the choicer examples), but also serious novels painted the same picture of a Socialist Britain in which Attlee's henchmen and the spivs and wideboys of the black market were one and the same: 'The nine o'clock train to Paddington ... started five minutes earlier, and got in ten minutes later, than before the war. But then, in the intervening period, there had of course been a revolution' (Henriques 1951:339), wrote Robert Henriques lugubriously in his book *Through the Valley*, winner of the James Tait Memorial Prize for the best novel of 1950, which purported to portray a Britain in which the decline of the landed gentry, living pitiably off capital, was the paradigm of a grim new world:

'Go on then, Walter, balance the account. Put all your little knick-knacks on to one side of the ledger; load it with your free spectacles and wigs, your few shillings saved on food your uneconomic rents for houses that haven't been built. And on the other side put the rackets you've created; put the impossibility of saving an ... honest penny against your old age; of gettin' any reward for bright ideas or hard work ... tell us about ... the men who used to be queuein' for work and are now queuein' for a gamble on the dogs. And their wives who have to queue for six-pennorth of meat ... There's a way round every queue ... All you've done old boy, is to change the queues and change the people who find the way round them.'   (Henriques 1951:368–69)

This bitter class hatred seems paranoiac indeed when set against the mild reformism that was the Labour government in office. Social democracy in action was hardly revolution (Miliband 1969, 1973). Commited to full employment and to a programme of welfare reform, the Labour government was also associated with the redistribution of wealth, both as between individuals by means of taxation and on a collective scale by the nationalization of industry. What actually happened was that the government succeeded both in maintaining full employment and in improving Britain's economically weakened condition, increasing productivity and exports quite dramatically (Pollard 1969). But in so far as a redistribution of wealth occurred at all, it appears not to have touched the poorer sections of the community, but to have been restricted to within the bourgeoisie (Milward 1971). The Welfare State was also wrongly believed to have brought about a redistribution of wealth, but insurance contributions redistributed wages within the working class – from the young to the retired, or from the healthy to the sick. The flat-rate contribution operated as a regressive tax; it would be a larger proportion of a poor man's than of a rich man's income and therefore would represent a heavier burden on the low-paid worker. Tax allowances also benefited the rich more than the poor, since the low-paid might pay little or no tax to begin with. In addition, management executives and professional workers enjoyed all sorts of invisible, often untaxed benefits, 'top-hat' retirement schemes, the firm's car, preferential mortgage schemes and so on (Titmus 1962; Atkinson 1974).

Government planning and state expenditure tended to expand after the war, and:

'the government soon got into the habit of at any rate trying to control private investment and consumption as well as its own expenditures, in the interests of economic stability ... The crucial point was that changes in taxation and government expenditure were made not with an eye to balancing the budget but in the interests of the government's overriding objectives of which full employment was one of the most important.' (Stewart 1971:212)

while as early as 1948 Stafford Cripps introduced an incomes policy which tied wage increases to increased productivity, a dominant preoccupation in post-war capitalist society, ensuring that workers shall get a larger slice only of a larger cake. The *White Paper* on the subject of incomes policy stated quite frankly:

> 'It is essential that there should be no further general increase in the level of personal incomes without at least a corresponding increase in the volume of production ... Such an increase ... can only have an inflationary effect. Unless accompanied by a substantial increase in production, it would drive up prices and charges, adversely affect pensioners, children and other recipients of social services benefits, increase the money costs of our exports and so reduce their saleability, and by black market pressure make it almost impossible to operate the controls necessary in view of the continuing scarcity of supplies and manpower.'   (Beveridge 1950:4)

so that Beveridge was not alone in voicing his fear of inflation as the greatest threat to economic stability in a full employment economy.

Welfare reforms, just as much as the nationalization of the mines and the railways, actually facilitated the smoother running of the capitalist economy, and were in no way in conflict with the interests of power groups in private industry, so that on the whole they were tacitly if not openly welcomed, even by many in the Conservative Party, as improving the chances of industrial and social peace, just as the expanding schemes of factory welfare and personnel management raised productivity. The welfare reforms of the 1940s were not particularly dramatic, whether considered in themselves, or by comparison with other West European countries, yet they were greeted as an essential part of the 'socialism' that was supposed to have been born, and continued for many years to be described as 'revolutionary'. Yet before the war, as has already been suggested, there had been no particularly marked ideology of the Welfare State in Britain, nor had we been pioneers in the field. The change was surely due to political considerations. The desire of the Labour government to give the appearance of running a socialist economy while in practice maintaining a capitalist one, the role of the powerful yet entirely reformist labour movement and the investment of the dominant classes in social peace and the post-war settlement made an ideology of socialism achieved extremely useful.

Even today, however, it comes as a shock to read the actual words of the *Beveridge Report*, one of the most crudely ideological documents of its kind ever written. If this was socialism, then it was socialism with an authoritarian face indeed. But in fact the principles underlying the Report were not those of socialism, but were the principle of insurance; the principle of the subsistence income; and the principle of the sanctity of the family.

Beveridge did not envisage his scheme as being sufficient in itself to abolish want; for this to be achieved full employment and adequate wages were also required. It was an essential part of:

> 'a comprehensive policy of social progress ... Social Security is an attack upon Want. But Want is only one of five giants on the road of reconstruction and in some ways the easiest to attack. The others are Disease, Ignorance, Squalor and Idleness.'   (Beveridge Report 1942:7)

Clearly the 1944 *Education Act*, the setting up of the National Health Service, and the attempt to solve the housing problem were necessary adjuncts to the Beveridge scheme, but Beveridge himself was essentially concerned with income maintenance, and explicitly stated that 'The abolition of Want requires a double redistribution of income, through social insurance and by family needs'. He did not, therefore, commit himself to a redistribution of wealth from one class to another, nor did he envisage a change in the distribution of family income.

To achieve the sort of redistribution he was proposing, he put forward proposals of four kinds; the national insurance scheme, consisting of retirement pensions, widows' benefits, sickness, industrial injury and unemployment benefit, maternity grants and benefits, and the death grant; the supplementary benefits scheme, seen as a residual and diminishing 'safety net'; family allowances; and various tax relief schemes. The Report (pp. 11–12) stresses the moral advantages of a contribution scheme:

> 'Benefit in return for contributions rather than free allow-

ances from the State, is what the people of Great Britain desire. This desire is shown both by the established popularity of compulsory insurance and by the phenomenal growth of voluntary sickness insurance etc. It is shown in another way by the strength of popular objection to any kind of means test. This objection springs not so much from a desire to get everything for nothing, as from resentment at a provision which appears to penalise what people have come to regard as the duty and pleasure of thrift, of putting pennies away for a rainy day.'

The subsistence income, or floor, to be built by these contributions was however set so low, that the supplementary or non-contributory sector, which Beveridge expected to fade away, and saw as a measure to tide over those who had not been insured in the past, has on the contrary grown with the years. The subsistence level recommended by Beveridge was based on the work of Seebohm Rowntree (1936) who had tried to measure poverty scientifically by establishing a poverty line which calculated the minimum amount of money on which an individual could survive without malnutrition. This minimum was not intended as an actual guide line to decide a minimum income in the real world, since it was based on theoretical nutritional principles and made no allowances for social needs nor for actual eating patterns. But Rowntree was drafted on to the sub-committee that worked on the setting of actual benefit levels, and cannot be absolved from responsibility in the setting of these at a level that was actually below subsistence. All the 'social sundries' for which Rowntree had allowed in his surveys were cut out, and by the time the first benefits began to be paid in 1948 the cost of living had risen so that the benefits actually paid represented only 75 per cent of Beveridge's minimum in real terms and therefore an even smaller percentage of Rowntree's original irreducible minimum. It was therefore inevitable that National Assistance (later Social Security) benefits, far from withering away, were increasingly relied on. A second reason for growing reliance on supplementary benefits was the way in which women were defined by the *Beveridge Report*.

In so far as the Welfare State was initiated by the *National*

Insurance Act of 1946, following the Report, it never even intended to treat women equally. While anomalies were ironed out, so that, for example, the insurance of the single working woman would henceforth be treated in the same way as the single working man, yet her national insurance contribution was still to be lower than a man's, on the grounds not that her earnings were likely to be lower, but that a man has a family to support. Married women were not accorded even this degree of autonomy. Beveridge's Report throughout stressed the importance of the family as an economic unit; man and wife really are one person (p. 49):

> 'In any measure of social policy in which regard is had to facts, the great majority of married women must be regarded as occupied on work which is vital though unpaid, without which their husbands could not do their paid work and without which the nation could not continue. In accord with facts the Plan for Social Security treats married women as a special insurance class of occupied persons and treats man and wife as a team.'

The married woman was to be treated as befitted her legal status; as the dependant of a man and as entitled to economic support by him, both for herself and for their children (p. 50):

> 'During marriage most women will not be gainfully employed. The small minority of women who undertake paid employment or other gainful occupations after marriage require special treatment differing from that of a single woman. Since such paid work will in many cases be intermittent, it should be open to any married woman to undertake it as an exempt person, paying no contributions of her own and acquiring no claim to benefit in unemployment or sickness. If she prefers to contribute and to requalify for unemployment and disability benefit she may do so but will receive benefits at a reduced rate.'

This was justified by the argument that a married woman's need for benefit would be lower because expenses were shared with her husband (but as Barbara Wootton (quoted by Land 1971) pointed out this would also apply to single people living with parents or other workers of their own age); by the argument that her earnings were more likely to be interrupted by sickness than a single woman's (but this was true of any low-paid worker, yet there was no suggestion that all lower paid workers should get a lower rate of benefit); and by the argument that her working life would be interrupted by pregnancies. Reproduction was thus tacitly defined as a disability. Defined as a worker, the woman was less satisfactory because of her need to have time off for childbearing; and this has been the predominant post-war definition of woman's 'dual role', a negative one that sees her mothering function as interfering with her work, and her work function as interfering with her child rearing.

Beveridge in fact, proposed a special maternity benefit which was to be 50 per cent higher than the normal unemployment or disability benefit; to offset this: 'On grounds of equity a proposal to pay lower unemployment and disability benefit to married women is right in view both of the special maternity benefit proposed and of the general balance of contributions and benefits' (p. 44). (This proposal was implemented in 1948, but only survived until 1953, since when maternity benefit has been paid at the same rate as a man's unemployment or sickness benefit.) This proposed reward for maternity was of a piece with the moral basis for Beveridge's proposals for family allowances (p. 154) (actually implemented by the Coalition government in 1945):

'Children's allowances can help to restore the birthrate both by making it possible for parents who desire more children to bring them into the world without damaging the chances of those already born, and as a signal of the national interest in children setting the tone of public opinion.'

Beveridge, that is, was a good Imperialist, dismayed, as many had been before him, by the falling birthrate, and therefore anxious to get women back into the home (p. 52):

'The attitude of the housewife to gainful employment outside the home is not and should not be the same as that of the single woman. She has other duties ... Taken as a whole the Plan for Social Security puts a premium on marriage in place of penalising it ... In the next thirty years

151

housewives as Mothers have vital work to do in ensuring the adequate continuance of the British Race and of British Ideals in the world.'

There was a clear moral bias in the way women were treated and discussed in the Report. Not only did Beveridge want to get women back into the home so that they could breed the Imperial race, he also wished to discourage immorality. So while widows were treated – relatively – with generosity, were able to enjoy a pension on the basis of their husbands' contributions, and were able to continue to draw this even if they returned to work, Beveridge recommended a separation allowance for deserted, separated, and divorced wives only if the marriage breakdown occurred through no fault of their own. Along with his conception of the married state as one of dependence for women on their husbands, he accepted the doctrine of the guilty and innocent parties in marriage breakdown; these two assumptions created difficulties in trying to provide income support for deserted wives that Beveridge was unable, in the end, to surmount. No provision for unsupported mothers was included in the scheme as it became law, and large numbers of these women were thrown on the mercy of supplementary benefit. It was wrongly supposed that the numbers of these women with their children would remain insignificant just as it was wrongly supposed that most married women would not be working. These two incorrect predictions about life in post-war society have caused difficulties as regards insurance for women ever since. They are not, however, simply anomalies, or a hangover which could be righted by some kind of legal or economic juggling; on the contrary they stem from the central contradiction of the way in which women are defined by our society at every level – as dependants of their husbands. There was therefore a direct clash between the wife's right to maintenance, even if the marriage ended if it were through no fault of her own, and the insurance principle:

'Divorce, legal separation, desertion and voluntary separation may cause needs similar to those caused by widowhood ... If they are regarded from the point of view of the husband they may not appear to be insurable risks: a man cannot insure against events which occur only through his fault or with his consent; and if they occur through the fault or with the consent of his wife, his wife should not have a claim to benefit. But from the point of view of the woman, loss of her maintenance as a housewife without her consent and not through her fault is one of the risks against which she should be insured.'

(*Finer Report* Vol II 1974:140; see also Land 1976)

The cohabitation ruling, therefore, turns out only to be a particular instance of the general principle that women cannot be at one and the same time married, as we understand marriage, and independent. Therefore, the situation of unsupported mothers was unchanged by the *Beveridge Report*, and they were essentially in the same position as they had been under the *Poor Law*. It is true that the *1948 National Assistance Act* began with the historic: 'The Poor Law shall cease to have effect'; but the punitive element of the old *Poor Law* was in some sense retained, because benefits must induce shame and stigma if they are set at a level that reduces the claimant to abject poverty, and also because the insistence that unsupported mothers should in the first place look to their menfolk for maintenance led to punitive attitudes being retained in respect of their moral status and even today the Supplementary Benefits Commission retains the Victorian attitude towards the deserted wife, let alone the fallen woman, as a failed and degraded example of womanhood. There was even a discussion in the Beveridge Report as to whether unmarried mothers should receive maternity grant and maternity benefit; and although Beveridge concluded that they should, he sternly reminded his audience that: 'The interest of the State is not in getting children born, but in getting them born in conditions which secure to them the proper domestic environment and care' (p. 135).

Women's organizations did come out strongly against the Report's assumption of female dependency. Elizabeth Abbott and Katherine Bompass complained:

'The status given to the married woman in the report is not new, it is the reflection of her present status in law and insurance, that of a dependant without any right of her own person, by way of one penny of cash, though she doubtless can in both cases claim a legal right to subsistence ... It is with the denial of any personal status to the woman because she is married, the denial of her independent personality within marriage, that everything goes wrong.'

(Abbott & Bompass 1943:7)

but the women's efforts in petitioning the government to change this aspect of the Report were unsympathetically received, and Sir William Jowitt, Minister without Portfolio and later the first Minister of National Insurance, who received a deputation from the National Council of Women of Great Britain, described their demands as 'unreasonable' (*Finer Report* Vol II 1974:143). It was even suggested that a separation benefit might encourage marriage break-up.

Despite all this, it should be emphasized that Beveridge's views did not express an overt State conspiracy to get women back to the kitchen sink at the end of the war. To a great extent he simply reflected views commonly held at the time, and was not the only one to expect that, as before the war, marriage and work would continue to be alternatives for most women. It is true that nurseries were closed down at the end of the war, and soon fell back from their peak in 1944, when they were providing 72,000 places for children under two. After the war, the policy was adopted of providing nursery places only for children in cases of 'special need', but this reflected an attitude not so much towards the employment of married women as towards correct child care, stated in the Ministry of Health circular of 1945 (221/45) which set out the lines of the policy:

'The Ministers concerned accept the view of medical and other authority that, in the interests of the health and development of the child no less than for the benefit of the mother, the proper place for a child under two is at home with the mother. They are also of the opinion that, under normal peacetime conditions, the right policy to pursue would be positively to discourage mothers of children under two from going out to work; to make provision for children between two and five by way of nursery schools and nursery classes; and to regard day nurseries and daily guardians as supplements to meet special needs ... of children whose mothers are constrained by individual circumstances to go

out to work or whose home conditions are in themselves unsatisfactory from the health point of view, or whose mothers
are incapable for some good reason of undertaking the full
care of their children.'   (*Finer Report* Vol I 1974:458)

Many women did have to make way, at least for a time, for the
men returning from the Front: 'I am one of the many women
whose husbands have returned from the Forces, and who sud-
denly find themselves without the crowding activities forced
upon them during the war ... Now that I am solely a housewife again, I am finding life very quiet' (White 1970). Women's
lives appear to have been particularly drab during this
period. For the housewife the reality of life continued to be
shortages and queues and this was the more dispiriting since
Britain had supposedly been victorious in the war. Things even
got worse. In 1946 bread was rationed, and in 1947 the butter,
meat, and bacon rations were cut. Even the sweet ration was
halved. Other necessities such as soap powder, nappies, rubber
teats, and baby cereals, although not rationed were almost un-
obtainable. How could women do their job as wives and
mothers adequately when they lacked the material necessities?
Their situation was summed up by the make-up advertisement:
'It was a day for looking young and gay, but ... darling you
look tired, he said.' Their reaction was the opposite to that of
mothers after the First World War. Whereas then women had
emphasized their emancipation and rejected a return to hamper-
ing clothes, now women escaped the drabness by an adoption of
traditional femininity as symbolized by the New Look. The
Labour government tried to stem this tide of extravagance, but
the mood of nostalgia was irresistible and it was in vain that
prominent Labour women attacked the new fashion for its
'caged bird atitude' and its betrayal of women's new freedom.
These more politically aware women did perceive it as an attack
on female emancipation, but their arguments got unfortunately
mixed up with Crippsian austerity and labour movement
puritanism, and their protests were ineffective (Sissons and
French 1963).
    Yet those responsible for government economic policy ap-
proached the problem of the declining birthrate from a point
of view distinct from that of Beveridge; no more than Beveridge

was the New Look part of a conscious conspiracy to get women back into the home, and other influences were at work. During the war the Ministry of Reconstruction had commissioned a Report on the attitudes of women towards continuing to work after the war, on the assumption that they would continue to be needed. One of the clauses in the *1944 Education Act* was the removal of the marriage bar for women teachers; in 1945 the Civil Service abolished its marriage bar, and by 1947 one in five of all married women were working, ¾ million more than in 1939. The Economic Survey for 1947 stated that: ' "The need to increase the working population is not temporary, it is a permanent feature of our national life ... women now form the only large reserve of labour left and to them the Government are accordingly making a special appeal" ' (Land 1971 : 116). There were always two sides to the coin, and it was after the war that social workers definitively weighed in on the side of a traditional attitude towards women's role. *The 1948 Children Act* (the result of the Curtis Report on children in care) re-quired a reorganization of services hitherto under the *Poor Law* but now to be carried out under the auspices of the new Children's Departments; and this required in turn an expansion of social work and increased numbers of trained social workers. Their preoccupation with the importance of traditional family life was marked, as was the influence of psychoanalytic teach-ings on the growing profession. During the war – when Anna Freud (Freud and Burlingham 1974) was working with and writing about refugee children and children in residential care – the work of Freud in its application to children was more and more influencing social work, but hitherto social work with families and adults, and marital work, had been discussed in terms of friendship and moralism, so that a social worker towards the end of the war (when there was considerable anxiety about the supposed decline in sexual morals) could write of the serious problem of :

> 'the general slackness of public opinion on sex-relation-ships, the appalling casualness with which young men and girls pick each other up, in pubs, cafés, dance-halls or the streets, and the risks they run whilst feeling so pitiably cocksure ... Though the approach of the Moral Welfare Movement has always been on religious grounds, there seems

little trace during recent years of any organised crusade by the Churches against what is regarded by all demoninations as grave sin ... A regrettably large proportion of our people "leave school and religion at the same time", and – also regrettably – are more likely to be encouraged by their parents to attend evening classes than to practise their religious duties.'   (Anon. 1944:8)

Gradually the language of psychology completely replaced the language of religion and moralism. Social workers after the war were anxious to help in the rebuilding of family life. At times they described perceptively the difficulties faced by recently reunited families:

'In many families the father is still away and the mother is coping single-handed; in some families where the father has been killed, she will always have to cope single handed and it is a hard job for a woman who is working part of the day if not all the day, to clothe, feed and bring up her children. When the children have been evacuated, she has to get to know them again ... One of the most difficult tasks facing the social worker today is the rebuilding of family life after years of separation and strain ... Husbands are returning home to find that their wives are no longer the young immature girls they left behind. They have acquired new interests; many are suffering acutely from six years of anxiety – the result of bombing, evacuation, the anxious hours spent each day in queues and, most of all, from the strain of being the only parent in charge of difficult and unruly children. Much of this worry and trouble has been deliberately withheld from the husband. Letters have been cheerful; in many cases wives have not told of the destruction of their homes or of the serious problems which adolescent members of the family have brought. The shock to the returning husband is very great.'   (Astbury 1946:237–41)

It was partly because of these situations, peculiar to wartime, that post-war social work from the start identified its task as the support and rebuilding of traditional family life. A vulgarized version of Freud could be used both to argue for the reassertion of well-defined male and female roles and in an attack on the Welfare State itself:

'Unless the nurture of the child proceeds normally within the family circle up to the age of puberty, the natural weaning which then takes place, with the assumption of adult privileges and responsibilities, does not occur. There follows a tendency for the man or woman to retain towards society the infantile dependence appropriate in the child, with a demand for maintenance as a right without obligations in return. While the child is justified in this attitude the adult is not. The adult should contribute to society as much or more than he receives back. This may throw some light on the current blindness to the economic truth that society as a whole cannot spend more than it produces, as well as the growth of totalitarian societies notable for their infantile characteristics.'   (Maberley 1948 : 164)

So the social worker's job of bolstering up the nuclear family could even become part of the Cold War struggle against communism. More generally, the return of the father ushered in a new paternalism and conservatism at this very time of the supposed creation of the 'socialist' Welfare State.

This period then saw the development of a contradiction between the need to expand the labour force, and the need to raise the birthrate, and tangling with this were new anxieties about the emotional well-being of children. Women have been the battleground of this conflict within capitalist society ever since, for what has been attempted is to retain the mother as, in practice, the individual solely in charge of the day to day care of children and yet at the same time to draw married women, the last remaining pool of reserve labour, into the work force. These demands are not fully compatible. Proof of their incompatibility are the many painful compromises to which women must resort, and the suffering to them and their families as a result.

EIGHT

Women & welfare: past & future

The critique of women's position when it came was in part a result of the very Welfare State that had been constructed on an assumption of their oppression. It was an unintended outcome of the expansion of higher education in the sixties, and also related to the generalized student revolt that came out of the universities. Student unrest was in part a response to the contradiction between the liberal pretensions of humanist education and the technological realities of the employment world and for women there was a special version of this contrast between the specious freedoms of academia and the reality of life afterwards.

Already in the early sixties a phenomenon known as the 'Observer Wife' had emerged. The women's pages of quality papers began to carry stories of housebound housewives and graduate mothers, women from that tiny elite of girls who had made it to university, but who five years later found themselves doing the same job of housework and child care as the girls who had left school at fifteen. Westergaard and Resler (1975) suggest that whereas a significant proportion of wives from the working-class have always worked, middle- and upper-class women did not fully begin to abandon the idea of 'marriage as a career' until the early 1960s. A national housewives register was set up through the columns of the *Guardian*, women were put in touch with one another, and groups formed; in some cases these must have been an ur-form of the consciousness-raising groups of the Women's Movement that began a few years later.

Women began to measure the ideology that told them they had achieved equality with the reality they were facing. Hannah Gavron's *The Captive Wife* (1968) summarized and brought out contemporary feeling accurately. There was the paradox of apparent achievement:

> 'Legally and politically women, apart from one or two minor points, are now equal to men ... In educational terms opportunities are not far short of those provided for men. Opportunities for work have greatly increased, particularly in some of the newer industries ... The status of women in relation to men has risen considerably. The number of roles which women can perform in society has increased and become more varied. Women have experienced an extension in the freedom of choice as to which roles they wish to perform.'
> (Gavron 1968:45)

Yet this left unanswered the bewildering question of why so few women were making their mark in the professions or industry, in Parliament or the Civil Service or even the Arts. This, in the sixties, when the wastage of educated and trained women in the workforce was more keenly felt than it had been in the fifties, had become a problem, with the emigration of trained men from this country. (Titmuss calculated that: 'Since 1949 the United States has absorbed – and to some extent deliberately recruited – the import of 100,000 doctors, scientists and engineers from developed and developing countries' (1967).) But it was not an economic problem only. The woman locked in the home appeared increasingly backward and at variance with the rest of capitalist society. The main body of Hannah Gavron's book was a survey of wives at home with young children, and she concluded from her interviews that to retire from work in order to have a family involved a loss of status for women, and a consequent sense of unimportance and loss of identity as well as loneliness. (These were working-class as well as middle-class women.) This led her to consider further the conflicting roles women have to play in modern society, and the stress this has caused. Yet her only solution, apart from more nursery facilities, was to suggest that community associations such as Parent Teacher Associations on the American model might integrate women more fully into community life, and that to further this re-integration transport and other facilities should be improved so that instead of being imprisoned at home, mothers with young children could take them everywhere with them – not a solution all mothers with toddlers would welcome. Her analysis, whilst clear and sympathetic, failed fully to expose the roots of the problem. In so far as she sought an explanation it appeared to be in terms of an historical hangover, a situation in which social institutions such as schools had somehow not caught up with a changed perception of women's capabilities. She did, however, point to the confusions surrounding women's sexual capacities, and while not making the breakthrough did appear to be reaching towards this – the area of sexuality – as the locus of the problem and its possible solution :

'The confusion over what constitutes the essential psychology of the woman is extended to equal confusion about what constitutes her sexual role. Freud (1932) considered this to be in part a passive one. He also felt that the sexual instinct in women was less strong than in men. Yet our society is by no means certain that women have or indeed should have weaker sexual desires. Until very recently, a popular view was to conceive of two types of women, virtuous and vicious. This was the accepted view in the nineteenth century and it was against just this type of mentality that Josephine Butler waged her campaign against the Contagious Diseases Act. The Act has long since been repealed but the ambivalence is still with us, although today the same respectable woman is often required to play both roles. Thus as Clifford Kirkpatrick (1955) says, women are asked to show restraint premaritally ... but afterwards – in marriage – she is expected to be ardent and uninhibited.'

(Gavron 1968 : 129)

The coming together, therefore, of two aspects of women's oppression in the sixties made possible the beginnings of the Women's Liberation Movement. Disappointed expectations in the wake of higher education (after graduating many young women found they still had to take a secretarial course or further vocational training) and a more sophisticated level of sexual exploitation combined with the political experience of the late sixties to awaken a new sense of frustration and rebellion amongst women, especially in those on the Left who found that the revolutionary ideals of their men did not prevent them from despising women.

The growth of the Women's Movement over the past seven years has made a great impact on British society. No doubt this has been one of the reasons that both Tory and Labour Governments have sought to meet certain feminist demands by bringing forward legislation to deal with equal pay and sex discrimination, laws that represent more than either a concession or an attempt to buy off protest. They reflect also a real tension as to what is required of women. For in the current crisis the contradictory pressures on women become sharper rather than lessening.

In a recent article Jean Gardiner (1975) has examined the two arguments put forward by Marxists to explain women's position in the labour force. Are they a reserve army of labour, drawn into work in times of boom and expelled during a slump? Or are they a cheap labour force likely to be used as substitute cheap labour for men during a period of crisis? Female unemployment is harder to calculate than that of men since the majority of married women (nearly two thirds of the female labour force at the present time) are not insured in their own right, do not qualify for unemployment benefit, and therefore do not bother to register as unemployed. However, Jean Gardiner suggests that unemployment among both men and women has grown in roughly equal proportions. There is also further hidden unemployment among women who would seek work if they were able to find adequate day care for their children. Audrey Hunt (1968) pointed to this as far back as 1965 in the Government survey of women's employment. There has been no expansion of nursery care. Yet the number of women employed rose by about 600,000 between 1966 and 1974 while the number of male employees throughout the economy declined by nearly $1\frac{1}{4}$ million, so that as a proportion of the total working force women have risen from 37 to 40 per cent (Gardiner 1975). This increase has been within the service and public sector, which have in any case been the growth sectors of the economy since the end of the Second World War. Women have not on the whole been substituted for men, but on the contrary, areas of men's work and of women's work have remained segregated. Jean Gardiner also suggests that women are more likely to be made redundant than are men. This is because they are often employed in a part-time or temporary capacity, which means that employers are not bound to pay them redundancy grants under the 1965 Act. On the other hand women often find it easier to get alternative employment and are more readily reabsorbed into the labour force than are men. They remain a cheap source of labour since at present their average earning capacity is at most sixty per cent of that of men. Nor are they a highly unionized workforce; about 32 per cent of women workers are unionized, about 27 per cent of the total working force, and although their numbers in the unions are growing they lack representation in the union hierarchy since only 2 per cent of paid TUC officials are women. In the context of the present crisis, cuts in state spending and welfare services may cut back on job availability as well as keeping more women in the home to tend sick and aged relations as well as children, but at the same time:

'Women workers, especially part-time workers, offer a number of advantages to employers who want to make a quick profit in an economic situation of long term crisis. In such a situation employers are unlikely to risk heavy investment in highly productive capital-intensive techniques of production which would enable them to employ a high-wage labour force. They are more likely to prefer processes requir-

ing a lot of cheap labour and relatively low capital investment. Women workers, and especially part-time workers ...
provide a suitable labour force in such circumstances, both
because they are relatively cheap in employment and because
they are more easily and more cheaply displaced when no
longer needed.'   (Gardiner 1975:14)

The solution of part-time work, often promoted as progressive by liberals and undersigned by both political parties,
whether in the *Plowden Report* (1967) or in Mrs Thatcher's later
proposals, can only be a solution for capitalism, not for women.
This is not only because part-time workers are a vulnerable
section of the work force. It is also because there is an unspoken
and *false* assumption that part-time work for women ensures the
adequate care of their children. It is assumed that part-time
workers are women with school age children and that their
work hours fit in with school hours; but this is by no means
always the case. Even if the children have reached school age
the mother's day must include tiring journeys with children to
school both before and after work, and anxiety if she is late or
the children unwell. There is still the problem of the school
holidays. In any case many children of working mothers are
below school age and likely to be left with child minders. Often
the only solution is the evening shift. Although too it is often
assumed that men now help with the housework, research
(Central Statistical Office 1974; Young and Willmott 1973) recently carried out shows that they still do less than half the
amount of housework done by women at work, and moreover
even when their help is considerable it is still the woman in
the household who carries the overall responsibility for the
organization of housework and the smooth running of the
household in most cases. The lot of working-class women,
therefore, is likely to continue to be low-paid low-skill work
and super exploitation.

At the other end of the social scale the picture is rather different, yet in some ways similar. The possibility of higher education has meant that there are women in most professions.
There are however very few in 'top jobs'. Only 3 per cent of
the members of the Institute of Directors are women. 25 per
cent of housemen (junior doctors in hospitals) are women, but

only 7 per cent of consultants, while of that 7 per cent most are in either the traditionally women's specialisms of paediatrics and child psychiatry, gynaecology and obstetrics, or in less prestigious sectors such as adult psychiatry and geriatrics. In teaching, at the basic grade of assistant teacher, women outnumber men by three to one; but there are more men than women heads of primary schools; and six times as many male as female heads of comprehensive schools (these figures refer to 1969). The same trend is found in social work where out of nearly 200 Directors of Social Services departments only 14 were women in 1972. Yet whereas equal pay for unskilled female workers remains a dream, in the spheres in which, theoretically, women already have equal pay and where the old disabilities such as the marriage bar have gone, there is some real desire to smooth the way for women who want to pursue a career. Yet here too the contradiction still remains between women's work at home and their work outside the home.

Attempts have been made at the ideological level to deal with this. There has been a – limited – move away from rigid gender-role indoctrination since the fifties. Bowlby, and the worries about latchkey children, did not actually stop working-class women from going out to work; they had to, they needed the money. The women it *did* stop were the more highly skilled ones who were more vulnerable to the influence of Bowlby, made to feel guilty by the idea that they might be damaging their children if they went out to work, and, if highly intelligent, still imbued with the fear that this would make them unattractive to men, for even in the fifties the psychology of the surplus woman was still deeply ingrained. Yet these were precisely the women the economy more and more needed.

In the fifties educationalists, politicans, social workers, and women themselves had believed the Bowlby myth. It was not simply a conspiracy to keep women in the home. It was the result of genuine anxiety, and it was genuinely hoped that efforts to improve family life would be successful. Instead it became clear that the discontent of many mothers who stayed a home – in order not to feel guilty of neglect, but who then experienced a new source of guilt in their dissatisfaction with the narrowness of their lives – might lead to even more problems. There was no decline in delinquency, as measured by crime statistics, and in the late sixties student radicalism was linked with permissive and over involved mothering (see the latest edition of Spock's manual on baby care, in which there is a new (or renewed) emphasis on discipline).

A more flexible approach to family roles was needed. As early as 1959 E. M. Goldberg, an influential social work researcher, undertook a study which showed her – what most of us know – that the lives of individual families frequently do not conform to a stereotype:

'There is no sharp division between the normal and abnormal, but rather a spectrum ... neurotic symptoms, oddities and unconventional role assignments need not necessarily lead to unhappy families or severely maladjusted children so long as the members of the family can play roles which help to fulfil their own as well as the needs of others in the family and as long as there is some capacity to tolerate individual differences and some sharing of common values. Only when emotional instability is combined with incompatability between the parents and conflicting values, does the family cohesion and the mental health or their members seem seriously threatened. (Younghusband 1965:26)

Yet this statement of the obvious constitutes in its context an ideological statement and a message to influential groups of social workers that a new sophistication was needed to achieve the preservation of the family, which remained the goal for social work. The maintenance of family life in a new situation was also the goal of a massive research project set up in the late sixties by the Leverhulme Trust and PEP, to explore the possibility of a more diversified family life. The authors of the book which came out of the project were helped by the Human Resources Centre of the Tavistock Institute of Human Relations, and the purpose and hopes of their study were clear:

'The case for careers for highly qualified women at a level commensurate with their abilities, and on an equal footing with men, can be argued on several grounds; personal interest and family need, civil rights, or, more cold-bloodedly, the need of the economy to use its biggest reserve of untapped ability.' (Fogarty, Rapoport, and Rapoport 1971:18)

Their study was of 'dual-career' families, where both parents work, which, they suggested (p. 18):

> 'are particularly interesting for the way in which they are pioneering ... a style of living which combines full participation for the wife as well as the husband in high-level employment together with the maintenance of the traditional values of family life.'

It is clear from their work that the dual-career families they describe also require the maintenance of a traditional class structure in order to function; women of the professional class who successfully combine career and motherhood almost invariably depend on an assortment of – female – servants, so that the emancipation of these women depends very directly on the continued exploitation of their working-class sisters, not infrequently women from underdeveloped countries.

In the United States (Cloward and Piven 1973) this has perhaps been more marked. The programme of Aid to Families with Dependent Children (AFDC) and the 'welfare explosion' in the sixties led to militant welfare workers acting to get more mothers on to the rolls, and discouraging them from taking the menial jobs which were all they could get. This in turn led to a backlash and an intervention from President Nixon himself. Having extolled menial work as more dignified than dependence on welfare, he went on:

> 'Domestic help has been difficult or impossible to obtain for many years, with – according to some estimates – several millions of jobs going begging. As a result, millions of our college-educated women cannot use their talents to pursue the professional careers for which they have been trained, and must spend much of the rest of their lives as chambermaids, cooks and cleaning women.' (Weinberger 1975:250)

This is the baldest possible statement of the drive to split the professional minority of privileged women from the rest who are *not* too clever and talented to be cooks, chambermaids and cleaning women (see also Ellis and Petchesky 1972).

Even more interesting than the economic implications of the dual-career family study was the need felt by its authors to reassure their readers – or themselves – about the direction in which their work pointed:

> 'Men and women ... will not cease to be men and women in the process. One of the most significant findings of the family studies reported here is that dual-career and similar patterns do not imply masculine women or feminine men, any more than they need imply any disadvantage to children. Past views on this have been biased by the fact not only that those women who fought their way through the barriers of discrimination to reach top positions had often to be exceptionally tough ... but also that so many of the women who reached these positions hitherto have been single ... The present studies have paid special attention to married men and women, and in their case no necessary or even probable correlation appears between a wife having a career and the feminisation of men or the masculinisation of women.'
>
> (Fogarty, Rapoport, and Rapoport 1971:18)

Like Beveridge, these writers, the Rapoports, are 'revolutionaries' finding 'radical' new ways to harness the family group more willingly to the service of capitalism. That is not to say that they are doing this consciously; they simply operate from an unquestioning assumption of capitalism and the modern family as the only possible economic and social forms. Naturally, they are anxious to make it all work better. Yet their insistence on the continuance of 'masculinity' and 'femininity' strikes a slightly hysterical note in an otherwise academic study, and it is indeed interesting that they feel so anxious about this, when they *are* prepared to criticize the nuclear family and traditional roles:

> 'Because men have tended to be economic providers and women have cared for infants, it is argued that babies need their mothers and that men need to be breadwinners. Because the nuclear family has been in recent times the basic form of social organisation, it is assumed that it is the form best adapted to modern society. Because more men are ambitious and committed to work in contemporary society than are women, it is argued that this is the way men and women basically are ... This essentially conservative view ... does

not take into account the emergence of new ecological conditions, never before known, which call forth new structural forms which have not been recorded or analysed.'

(Rapoport and Rapoport 1971:15)

Yet although aware that the woman locked in the home is
increasingly anomalous, these authors lack the courage to take
the final step of questioning consciousness, or what some psychologists and social workers like to call 'identity'. It is no
doubt for the same reason that while society is beginning to
accommodate itself to those demands of the Women's Movement that centre round economic improvements, and while
population policies are urged, there remains an intense ambivalence on the questions of abortion and sexual activity outside
marriage. The more far-reaching reconsideration of sexuality
and thus of consciousness attempted by some women generates
the fury and anger born of pure fear. Lesbianism and female
aggression are experienced as a major assault on the integrity
of the bourgeois personality.

This is one reason women still fear to make demands for
themselves. If they do want to achieve, they feel they have to
do so 'as men' yet retain their femininity at the same time. A
Financial Times report of a meeting of women executives at the
British Oxygen Company illustrates this attitude:

'The meeting was quite free of any strident complaints
about inequality and the general unfairness of life to women.
Suggestions that the company should run a creche or in some
other way make allowances for women with children came
very low on the list of priorities ... The general conclusion
to be drawn from this meeting is that working women are
less preoccupied with their domestic problems, children,
husbands and housework than might be expected. They are
concerned about training and job opportunities and already
felt equal – but wanted acknowledgement of this equality.'

(2.7.1974)

(The reporter was also a woman.) The more privileged, in other
words, a woman is, the more difficult it is for her to understand either the privileged nature of her freedom, or its limi-
tations. One danger of the present situation is of a split

between working-class women and a minority of professional women, the articulate and trained women, who could be bought off at the expense of the majority. Yet one aspect of the dual role operates against this. Audrey Wise (1972) has suggested that one reason for female apathy about equal pay is that women workers have seen how men in exchange for high wages have accepted gruelling conditions of work, productivity deals, and increased exploitation in all its forms, and do not themselves wish to pay this price. Women tend more to raise issues related to the social conditions of work, adequate canteen and toilet facilities, rest periods, and child care provision. Equally women employed in the professions tend to seek work they enjoy and are not necessarily so anxious to reach the heights of the profession as are men. There are many reasons for this, including economic need and socialization, but it means that women can be a progressive influence within the unions. The *Equal Pay* and *Sex Discrimination Acts* offer opportunities for struggle that will keep to the forefront the situation of the more exploited women in the economy. The fight for the acceptance of the Working Women's Charter over the past two years has led to new issues being raised in the unions, as has the fight against restrictive abortion legislation in 1975–76. And this heightened consciousness amongst many women in the labour movement must lessen the possibility of a split along class – in the sociological rather than Marxist sense – lines.

The British Welfare State has been copiously discussed since its beginnings. Its impact on the family, its impact on the working class, sometimes its impact on the middle class, have been examined, and there has been frequent discussion of its relationship to socialism. What has never been discussed is its impact on women. Yet women are central to its purposes, and it has always cast its safety net around the housewife and mother in her home. Even the feminist pioneers seem for the most part to have perceived their work as an effort to enable women more happily to undertake motherhood by being freed from economic and social stress.

This should not cause surprise or blanket condemnation, for, as R. M. Titmuss (1963) pointed out, it is only during the last fifty years that the average span of women's lives has reached much beyond their child-bearing and child-rearing years. The contemporary Women's Movement represents one response to changing conditions (just as the Victorian feminists represented a reaction to changed conditions for women in their lifetime). Another reaction is seen in hesitant and fumbling gestures towards change amongst planners and employers. The dominant ideology of society responds as well. Social policies and family policies represent a response. To what are they now responding?

It has already been suggested that economic changes since the Second World War have affected women's lives and that the greater likelihood of married women to be working – or to need to work – places them in a particularly sharp contradiction. The present economic crisis makes life even harder for women, whether working or not, for they must work harder in the home to make the same money go further, and they must bear the brunt of slashed welfare provisions. Hospital patients prematurely returned home to convalesce, elderly parents denied meals on wheels or home helps, children on half-time schooling, unemployed husbands for that matter, all require more attention from Mother.

Other changes too are taking place in society that change family life and with this women's lives. The greater life expectancy of adults today and the much smaller family size have already been mentioned. It is also the case that today more men and women enter into marriage. Professor D. V. Glass has shown that:

'there has been a dramatic swing to higher probabilities of marriage and to consistently falling ages at marriage ... In all, the changes in marriage frequency and age since the 1930s have been of a magnitude unequalled in any other period since the beginning of civil vital registration, and probably in the past two or three centuries.'

(Finer Report Vol I 1974 : 26)

As he also pointed out, this has affected fertility because it means that a higher proportion of women is exposed to the risk of pregnancy for longer periods, and this has tended to reduce the frequency of childlessness, which is linked to late marriage. What has occurred has been a *compression* of fertility. Fewer women are childless, but more complete their families at an earlier age and within a short span of time. Thus, whereas in 1940, after ten years of marriage the average size of a woman's family would be 1.63 and she reached the average family size of 2.00 only after twenty-five years of marriage, in 1960 she had reached the figure of 2.13 after only ten years of marriage (*Finer Report* Vol I 1974). Some attempts have been made to discover the extent to which the falling age at marriage is related to social class, and there is some evidence – although little is known about the subject – that this is the case; amongst the brides of unskilled workers 20 per cent were marrying in their teens in the years 1947 to 1951, but 41 per cent in 1960 to 1961; amongst brides of skilled workers the proportion was 19 per cent in 1947 to 1951 and 32 per cent in 1960 to 1961. The proportions of teenagers marrying men from the class of employers, managers or self-employed professionals were low, nor did they show a significant increase over the same period (*Finer Report* Vol I 1974). Here might be found a basis for the split, discussed above, between working-class and middle-class women. The horizons of the educated expand while those of the working-class girl remain confined to romance, marriage, and children, since these are the only available tokens of status and maturity. At the same time, the decline in family size affects all classes.

These demographic changes have certain consequences for family life. They suggest that more women – and men – wish to have the experience of parenthood, but that women particularly no longer wish to devote the larger part of their lives and identities to motherhood. In the light of these facts Mia Kellmer Pringle's fashionable and widely canvassed views on the maternal role (*The Times* 14.1.1976) (and see above Chapter Five) would seem to be in conflict with what women actually want.

The setting up of the Finer Committee in 1969 did in fact reflect a generalized anxiety about marriage breakdown in our society. The Report suggested that there was cause for anxiety in that it calculated the number of one-parent families at 620,000: 'Nearly one-tenth of all families with dependent children have only one parent by reason of death, divorce, separation or births outside marriage ... nearly two-thirds of a million parents are looking after one million children single-handed' (Vol II: 78), and this means that over a period of time the number of children who at some stage have been in single-parent families will be much larger, although there is little information on rates of remarriage, marriage or subsequent cohabitation amongst lone parents. The largest group is of deserted wives and their children (not of mothers who were never married). Moreover, further anxiety has been felt in official quarters of late at the apparent increase in family violence. Whether it is an actual increase that has resulted in a number of deaths of children at the hands of one or other parent is not clear. Nor is it clear that more women today are battered than was previously the case. It may well be that tolerance towards violence of both kinds within the family has diminished. Certainly both kinds of violence were frequent and well-documented in Victorian times (Pinchbeck and Hewitt 1973). Renewed concern today has arisen in the case of children because of the adverse publicity given to a number of recent cases which caused embarrassment to local authorities. These have a statutory duty to prevent child neglect and to care for the deprived and abused child. One result of several enquiries into non-accidental child deaths has been that social workers of local authorities have become readier to receive children into care, and there is a changed emphasis away from the importance of the child–mother tie, to be preserved at all costs, towards the neglectful mother, seen in a punitive light. For example, in a recent case, that of Steven Meurs, while the official investigation report bent over backwards to exonerate the social worker (a young woman, who was however accused of 'identifying too closely' with the mother, that is of being too friendly and sympathetic), it described Mrs Meurs as 'cold and heartless'. Yet Mrs Meurs was aged only 20, was being treated for depression by her GP, and had on one occasion taken an overdose. She was also 'coping with an unsettled marriage, a husband in prison and various men friends' as well as her own two children. On top of this the local authority allowed her to keep four children of her aunt, taken in by Mrs Meurs after a marital dispute (the *Guardian* 16.1.1976). It is appropriate to point out here that recent research (Brown 1974) has suggested that young mothers at home with children tend to suffer from depression and do not find their lives satisfying in many cases.

The attitude of local authorities and officialdom towards

battered women has also changed, but for other reasons. They have no statutory duty to protect women and there has been great reluctance to acknowledge the existence of a problem at all. Social workers, trained to support family life, have tended to perceive the problem of the battered woman as simply an extreme manifestation of a neurotic marriage relationship and the couple as immature, disturbed, or 'deprived' individuals in need of counselling, therapy, and support rather than separation (NSPCC 1974), particularly as that would involve more provision of the costliest resource of all – housing, and possibly the reception of children into care, while the man may be made homeless. In the past (and it happens still) a beaten woman was usually told by local authority housing or homelessness sections that she could not be registered as homeless because she had a home – in other words she could be compelled to return to the man who had abused her. A similar attitude appears still to be rather common in the police force today. For example, the evidence submitted to the Select Committee on Violence in Marriage, set up in 1975, by the Association of Chief Police Officers of England, Wales, and Northern Ireland, stated that (p. 366):

'Whilst such problems take up considerable Police time during say, 12 months, in the majority of cases the role of the Police is a negative one. We are, after all, dealing with persons "bound in marriage", and it is important, for a host of reasons, to maintain the unity of the spouses.'

The attitudes of social workers and local authorities has to a certain extent moved more towards one of pity for these women as rather pathetic and inadequate victims. This has followed the setting up of Chiswick Women's Aid by Erin Pizzey, who was successful in attracting much publicity for the problem of wife-beating. Subsequently many other women's refuges began to open. By October 1975 the National Women's Aid Federation (see Weir and Hanmer 1976) (to which Erin Pizzey does not belong) counted fifty member groups operating thirty-five houses. For the most part these groups were started by women's groups subscribing more or less closely to the aims and ideals of the Women's Movement, although in some groups social workers have been to the fore. Many have – after a struggle –

been supported by their local authorities, sometimes with money, sometimes with housing, and although some authorities have refused to give any help the more canny have realized that by supporting a women's refuge largely run on voluntary labour they may have found a cheap solution to an embarrassing problem, and perhaps also defused possible protest on a larger scale. In times of economic crisis voluntary and self-help groups become popular with government, and this is a problem that must be faced by the Women's Movement when it operates in these ambiguous spheres on the uncertain border between social work and political activism. This ambiguity is not of course peculiar to Women's Aid, or indeed to the Women's Movement as a whole. The Claimants Unions (H. Rose 1972) were beset with it; Sylvia Pankhurst inevitably found herself engaged in sorting out welfare problems as part of her political work in the East End; while Doris Lessing (1966) describes a similar problem as she encountered it when engaged in political work as a Communist Party member in East Africa.

Social workers, and the State, are also faced with the breakdown of family functioning in the failure of the 1969 *Children and Young Persons Act*. This was intended to facilitate the supervision of juveniles brought before the courts, by family social workers, and the emphasis was to have been on a Seebohm approach to the whole family. This has failed for various reasons, among them being the shortage of social workers and the shortage also of institutions, where needed, as an alternative to the child's home. Its failure has shown how the family as an institution can no longer cope with – or at least can often no longer control – many older children and adolescents, a further symptom of the disintegration of the family.

One question we should ask then is: how is the State likely to cope with this disintegration? Equally important, what demands should we ourselves struggle for in this situation? On the other hand account must be taken of a second and contradictory aspect of modern family life; that by 1971 only 50 per cent of households consisted of families with children (unpublished paper by Jean Gardiner) – another effect of the compression of fertility. Among the 50 per cent of households where there are no children will be many old and single people fending for themselves. There will also be many couples, where the bulk of the housework will probably be done by the wife. This brings us back to the subject of housework, and prompts a further, and more general question: 'Why have housework and childcare, in modern industrial capitalist societies such as Britain, continued to such a great extent to be the responsibility of women and organised on a private family basis?' (Gardiner 1975:47).

Because more and more married women are going out to work, and because, although there has been a rise in the number of women who bear a child or children at some point in their lives maternity has become quantitatively less and less absorbing, the importance, drudgery, and significance of domestic work in the home has become more and more clear (Gardiner 1975). Why then is it retained? Why has it not been socialized when in the industrial sphere capitalism constantly seeks to transform and revolutionize its technology? The economic significance of domestic labour has been discussed for some years in the Women's Movement (e.g. Benston 1969; Morton 1970; Rowbotham 1973) and more recently the subject has been taken up by a number of socialists and Marxist economists (Harrison 1974; Secombe 1974). Whatever the precise nature of its relationship to surplus value it is clear that the domestic unpaid work of the housewife helps to keep costs down for the employer by making it possible for the worker to be cared for much more cheaply than would otherwise be possible. The socialized care of the worker – canteens, living accommodation, laundry – alone would be likely in this country to cost the capitalist more than the efforts of the housewife who takes pride in making do. Where it is cheaper for the workman to be separated from his family – as is the case in South Africa where black workers can be compelled to live in barracks – that is what happens. The strength of the working class has also much to do with the achievement of more tolerable living conditions.

There is a second reason for the retention of domestic work; the supportive emotional functions of the family. The intensity of the parental–child relationships within the family make for the vulnerability of the child and therefore the family is a highly functional ideological institution for the upbringing of children in such a manner that they conform, as adults, to authoritarian/submissive social relationships. Then there is the marriage relationship. It is pleasanter for workers to be married. The marriage relationship may have its problems, men may feel henpecked or hamstrung; the sexual relationship may have its inhibitions and disappointments, especially for the woman; yet State brothels could hardly provide an adequate substitute. And then, as the *Financial Times* with its usual perceptiveness has observed, the State looks to marriage and family life to calm the worker and turn him from a militant into a responsible citizen:

'The overall impression ... is that our population is becoming increasingly middle-class, with white-collar workers in the ascendancy and the family more firmly established than ever as the fundamental unit of what should be an extremely stable society ... The NEDC Report asserts bravely that "it is in their marriages and family lives that the majority of people in Britain find their most complete and enduring satisfactions ... One of the most important consequences of this change in the position of both the family and of women is that the demand for houses continues to grow ... between 1950 and 1972 the proportion of owner-occupied dwellings in the UK rose from 29 per cent to 51 per cent, one of the highest levels of owner-occupation in Europe." All those teenage couples want homes of their own ... The desire for a suburban residence is probably the strongest single economic force in Britain today.'   (18.6.1974)

The *National Economic Development Council Report* looked to the encouragement of more owner occupation as a form of 'levelling up' to be offered as an alternative to the redistribution of wealth, and to mute class divisions, while public housing should be reserved for the really poor and the homeless, seen as residual categories.

A third reason for the retention of the unwaged housewife and her children as the dependants of the individual worker is that this arrangement reinforces the incentive of the father to work regularly and hard. The ability to support a family is early equated in the male child's mind as an essential part of his manhood. Much value is attached to virility and loss of his job can lead to the man losing also his sense of identity in his own and his wife's eyes (see the *Guardian* 22.1.1976). The male role thus reinforces the work ethic quite directly.

These then are some of the reasons for the retention of domestic work within the nuclear family. And State Welfare provision has in practice increasingly meant the introduction of family policies, not only to bridge the gaps and repair the breakdowns, but also in a positive sense to promote desired forms of family care. Yet the post-war discussion amongst socialists of the Welfare State has largely ignored the development of family policies. At the time of its inception, Attlee's Welfare State appears to have been accepted by many on the Left as, if not true socialism, at least a significant step towards it. In the fifties Marxist debate of all kinds was muted, and it was not until 1958 that the *New Reasoner* published two articles which seriously attempted to evaluate the Welfare State. John Saville took the view that welfarism is a palliative that buys off revolt, and to illustrate the point gave the example of the phrase used by Joseph Chamberlain to explain his 'gas and water' socialism: 'What ransome will property pay for the security it enjoys?' (Saville 1958) and he argued that reforms such as the nationalization of coal did not mean at all the same thing in 1945 as they would have done in 1921. Dorothy Thompson on the other hand felt this view to be an over-simplified one that took no account of working-class struggles for social provision, and she saw certain provisions, in particular the NHS, as enclaves of socialism within the capitalist society (Thompson 1958). The view of Poulantzas (1973) which explains welfare spending as an economic concession to the working class both takes account of, and surpasses, these two interpretations. A view that takes account of the position of women must modify his view also, however, for if account is taken of family policies since the War as of employment policies after the First World War, then it becomes clear that the concessions have been mostly to the male half of the working class, and that where women were concerned there was an ideological attitude which continued to define them narrowly as wives and mothers at a time when they were increasingly seeking employment outside the home, and that welfare institutions have tended to express disapproval of and, not infrequently, to punish women who transgressed these norms. In practice family policies have in no way facilitated the 'dual' role of the working mother; rather this has been defined as a psychological problem. Social policies of all kinds have continued to define her and her children as dependants, until even bourgeois sociologists (Goode 1971) have had to admit that power is unevenly distributed within the nuclear family. Prestige, economic superiority, and the authority due ultimately to force to go the father, and it is only by her sexual attractions and her power to compel love and emotional dependency that the woman can hope to redress the balance. Effectively to use these, her only weapons, the woman must often appear manipulative and devious. In order to preserve the work ethic welfare policies have been put into practice which try to preserve a particular family form which is already beginning to break down; but this does not prevent employers from offering the kind of work that will draw women into the labour market, and their difficulties with family and children then create a fresh set of problems for the institutions that devise family policies. Thus is capitalism hoist on its own petard. As Anne Scott James said in 1945, the low birth rate is a women's revolt, today as then. There is the added factor that today women have found a new voice, they are supported by a political movement with a sophisticated and thoughtful analysis of the feminine dilemma. In the past, both here and in the Soviet Union, and today in certain socialist countries such as Czechoslovakia where legislation to discourage abortion was linked to concern at the low birthrate and possibly to employment problems as well, it has been possible to push women back into the home when this was convenient to the State. Whether it is still possible in Britain today is uncertain. If women continue to be needed in the labour force, despite high unemployment, and if their voice has become too loud to be ignored, then the State will be forced to search for new solutions to the old problem of child care, with results that are as yet impossible to foresee.

With the strings of the contradiction tightening, a new element has entered into the configuration during the past few years. Intensified class struggle has been particularly important within the white-collar sector. The increase in the number of state employees, civil servants at all levels, teachers, social workers, and technicians has led to an increase in the numbers and strength of their unions. Many of these workers are in fact a part of the Welfare State. These workers, although many of them have a 'middle-class' identification and some earn very high salaries, are 'proletarianized', that is, they are not self-supporting peasantry nor self-employed professionals, but they sell their labour in return for a wage (in this case from the State) like any worker. In recent years their rate of exploitation has increased. This means, for instance, that nurses have to work harder because patients are ejected from hospital at an earlier stage in their convalescence, so that the nursing staff deal with patients only at the height of their illness when they require more care, and simultaneously are deprived of the help about the ward of the patients who are getting better. Social workers, similarly, have bigger caseloads, with consequent alienation and heightened militancy. New 'techniques' of social work, such as 'crisis intervention' have been developed as justifications for social workers to spend less time with more clients, while traditional casework, which attempted to deal with problems in a more leisurely fashion approximating at times to psychotherapy, has fallen into disrepute. Teachers too, are at times, in the inner cities certainly, faced with the consequences of loss of social control and some do not survive the struggle to contain angry and frustrated adolescents of up to sixteen years old. In further and higher education, worsening staff–student ratios contribute to a poorer educational experience and cause discontent on both sides. No wonder that white-collar unionism has accelerated and that white-collar unions are now amongst the most militant. NALGO and NUPE for example led pay struggles in 1973 and 1974; and for the first time in many years struggles have included demands as to the nature and quality of social welfare care. 1974 saw auxiliary workers in hospitals take action over the continued existence of private beds and the use for their private patients by consultants of publicly financed hospital facilities. The T&GWU made successful demands for better pensions.

The questions of the control of welfare services and provision by those who use them and by the workers who staff them has also been raised. This is progressive and makes possible an integration of both economic (wage) demands and ideological demands. The fight to stop agency nurses being employed within the NHS for example was not only a fight to obtain better rates of pay within the health service, but also raised the whole question of the problems of the NHS and did also touch on the difficulties of the female labour force. Many of these strikes and protests have involved women in political battle for the first time, for after all women are a majority in many of these welfare services. Women have also been to the forefront of some of the battles for users' control; this has often arisen from their special position – which has usually weakened them in the past – as child-bearers. In relation to the NHS their special position has been particularly clear. Patients, men and women alike, are frequently treated as objects, as diseases rather than people. In many cases operations and forms of treatment are not properly explained, nor are patients given the opportunity to exercise a choice in full knowledge of the facts. Women are in a unique position to combat this because when pregnant they are not – theoretically at least (see Oakley 1975) – regarded as ill. The high status given to motherhood – again in theory – also comes into blinding conflict with the way women are often actually treated when giving birth in hospital, and the shock of being treated like one of a herd of cows – but no longer a sacred one – often gives women the strength to protest. Whereas a cancer patient, for instance, might understandably feel too frightened to do otherwise than acquiesce in whatever treatment is offered for his possibly painful or disgusting symptoms, a pregnant woman, although she does face danger, pain, and fear, is at least undergoing a known and comprehensible process and is not suffering from a malfunction. This is a strengthening factor, and collectively women today are beginning to demand the sort of care they themselves want when giving birth. They are demanding that the right be restored them of giving birth at home, if they wish. They are rebelling against false notions of pain in childbirth; either that the pain is intolerable only when the mother is psychologically badly adjusted to approaching motherhood, or alternatively that, being 'natural' the pain is somehow functional and must just be endured. They are rebelling against unnecessary inductions, 'daylight labour' and other rationalization processes in obstetric wards designed to cope with shortages of staff or supposed technological advance (Charlton and Muir 1975). In the case of abortion the particular position of women is even more clear. Here too, patients – women – who are not 'ill' are challenging the authority of the doctor by saying what *they* want, instead of meekly sitting back and accepting his diktat. This is one reason – although of course not the only one – that abortion is such a contentious issue.

I suggested earlier that the Women's Liberation Movement is a response to today's particular conditions in our society. It is of course more than that. It is the voice of an oppressed majority breaking through the silence that had engulfed them. It is a powerful revoluntionary political movement in the sense that it has necessarily raised ideological issues and has necessarily not confined itself to the trades union struggle (Lenin 1970). Its ideas are genuinely revolutionary in asserting the necessity of changed social relationships and while it is a part of the class struggle, and in essence spontaneously socialist (unlike its Victorian predecessor) it has also raised a new and possibly even more threatening issue in challenging sexism and the patriarchy – male power. The economism of the post-war Left (discussed in chapter 1), blind to the role of the State and of ideology, made it necessarily blind also to the sexism of our society. It was difficult for many socialists to admit that even in post-revolutionary societies the world over, sexism did not disappear overnight with the advent of socialism. Instead of the abolition of the family as it appears in bourgeois society, socialist countries have tended to retain it, or, where State provision has taken over some of its functions, these have tended to retain the paternalistic and authoritarian model of the patriarchal family (Weir, personal communication). (This is one of the reasons it has been difficult for the Women's Movement to discuss collective social and childcare provision in a way that is attractive – the available models of collective care are almost always patriarchal rule writ large, the large scale institution being the capitalist, and in particular the Victorian, giant-size version of the father-dominated family.) In Western European society the Left has spoken of the 'working-class family', yet within capitalist society working-class families are modelled on the bourgeois family, and within capitalism there can be no 'proletarian family' somehow free of the distortions of social relations under capitalism.

Engels stated what would be necessary before the emancipation of women could be even begun:

'The first premise for the emancipation of women is the reintroduction of the entire female sex into public industry; and ... this ... demands that the quality possessed by the individual family of being the economic unit of society be abolished.'
(Engels 1970:501)

Later he enlarged on this:

'The emancipation of women and their equality with men are impossible and must remain so as long as women are excluded from socially productive work and restricted to housework, which is private. The emancipation of women becomes possible only when women are enabled to take part in production on a large, social scale, and when domestic duties require their attention only to a minor degree. And this has become possible only as a result of modern large-scale industry, which not only permits of the participation of women in production in large numbers, but actually calls for it and, moreover, strives to convert private domestic work also into a public industry.'
(Engels 1970:569)

What later socialists have failed adequately to account for is why this process has not taken place in the rapid and extensive fashion Engels predicted. Only in writings from the recent Women's Movement has this been attempted, and the reasons, this study of welfare provision has suggested, are partly ideological, although the economic function of the privatized domestic work of the housewife is also of importance. Women are flowing into the labour force yet this has not led to the ending of the family in the way Engels imagined. For one thing, Engels never fully confronted the problem of child-rearing, and the determination of the bourgeois State to support and retain the family is closely connected with developing attitudes to child care.

The Women's Movement has, however, gone even further than this in suggesting that sexism and male dominance are even more deeply rooted than class divisions and perhaps originate from a different source. Feminists and socialists can agree with Engels when he identifies the first class antagonism

in history as coinciding 'with the development of the antagonism between man and woman in monogamous marriage, and
the first class oppression with that of the female sex by the
male' (Engels 1970:494). Monogamy represented a safeguard to
the property of the male. It is also possible to agree with Marx
and Engels when they say. 'The first division of labour is that
between man and woman for child breeding' (Engels 1970:464)
and with Engels when he elaborates upon this: 'Division of
labour was a pure and simple outgrowth of nature; it existed
only between the two sexes. The men went to war, hunted,
fished ... The women cared for the house, and prepared food'
(p. 567). However, whereas some socialists have argued that this
division of labour continues to be 'natural' at the present time,
feminists such as Shulamith Firestone (1971) have suggested
that modern technology today for the first time in history frees
women from their biological burden. Her assessment of the
possibilities of technology in present society is surely over-
optimistic, since after all, science is controlled by men; nor
does she acknowledge the necessity for changed social relationships if scientific knowledge is to be used to the advantage of
all members of society; yet she is surely correct to suggest that
ecological change and the possibilities of fertility control represent a crucial and qualitative change in women's position.

There are also points in Engels' text at which he appears to
take refuge in a view of women's nature typical of his age, that
is, when he seems to accept the belief in the greater refinement
and purity of the feminine nature. This seems to be the assumption of the following passage:

'The more the old traditional sexual relations lost their
naive, primitive jungle character, as a result of the development of the economic conditions of life, that is, with the
undermining of the old communism and the growing density
of the population, the more degrading and oppressive must
they have appeared to the women; the more fervently must
they have longed for the right to chastity ... This advance
could not have originated from the men, if only for the reason
that they have never – not even to the present day – dreamed
of renouncing the pleasures of actual group marriage.'

(Engels 1970:484–85)

Yet he then falls into the opposite error of idealizing proletarian sexual relations:

> 'Sex love in the relation of husband and wife is and can become the rule only among the oppressed classes, that is, at the present day, among the proletariat, no matter whether this relationship is officially sanctioned or not. But here all the foundations of classical monogamy are removed. Here, there is a complete absence of all property, for the safeguarding and inheritance of which monogamy and male domination were established. Therefore, there is no stimulus whatever here to assert male domination.'
>
> (Engels 1970:499–500)

Yet it is clear that male/female relationships in Victorian working-class Britain were often of the utmost brutality, and while Engels gives a passing mention to this, he dismisses it as a 'last remnant' of male domination. Today, male dominance while on the whole less brutal has become on the other hand more refined and is certainly psychologically as entrenched as ever.

The Women's Movement therefore has presented a challenge to traditional socialism, a challenge that has appeared the more threatening in that it has pointed a finger at the existence of sexism and male supremacy within the Left and the labour movement itself. It appears as even more challenging and threatening to the wider society, and has as a result been consistently distorted and misrepresented in the mass media. It is in fact a serious weakness of the Movement that its challenge has not been always coupled with a persistent political effort to gain broad-based support from the many emancipationist (see Wilson 1975 for a discussion of the distinction between women's emancipation and women's liberation) and progressive or partially progressive women's organizations. Support is growing amongst women trades unionists, but there is still a long way to go. Yet this weakness of the Women's Movement arises out of what is also a strength, that is, from its rejection of 'male' hierarchical structures and from a fear, too, that attempts to gain a voice within the mass media will only lead to a distortion or co-option of the message. Yet notwithstanding the initial horror with which Women's Liberation was greeted, it has already changed society and is becoming an ever stronger force for change.

Because its message has often been distorted, it seems necessary to conclude by restating it here, since any writing that challenges the family form is open to misrepresentation. I began by touching on the contradictory nature of the modern family as the locus of affection and emotion, but the place, at the same time, where women are subjected to the oppression of the State, and where the agent of that oppression is often an individual man. I should like to emphasize how difficult it is for all of us to imagine forms of personal relationship other than those we have, since our expectations have been structured by a process of continuous experience since birth. Many of us, therefore, feel personally threatened when the institution of the family is criticized and react as though this were a headlong attack on any form of loving relationship.

Yet when feminists challenge the adequacy of the nuclear family they do not – as is often suggested – attack the value either of continuous loving relationships for children or of emotionally satisfying relationships, in particular sexual relationships, for adults. They do not necessarily attack monogamy. Indeed, what the Women's Movement has to say on these matters is not ultimately an *attack* at all. It is an *analysis* of what is actually the case. It is an unmasking of reality. The Women's Movement points to the weakness of the family under capitalism. It remains an economic unit, but becomes an unstable one, because, whereas in pre-capitalist society all members of the family contributed directly and the family was a largely self-sufficient production unit, under capitalism this is no longer the case, and instead the economically weaker members of the unit, women and children, become more dependent on the man's higher wage than he is on their services. Thus the instability of the modern family, of which the *Finer Report* is both reflection and exposition, is an outcome of certain economic conditions. Historically too the family has received more social support of one kind or another than is the case today, and has not had to last so long, because life was shorter, and the Women's Movement therefore draws attention to a fact in indicating the unusually isolated nature of the nuclear family in present day urban society, and in particular the unusually isolated position of the woman within it.

There is nothing eternal, sacrosanct or even usual about the modern family. It has undergone a process of continual change; today, however, we are living through a period in which its atomization and disintegration have reached a point at which it seems problematic. The post-war contortions of the Welfare State have been in part an attempt to arrest this process.

What feminists, socialists, and all those who desire to see constructive changes in social relations, should seek are ways whereby social welfare care instead of trying desperately to shore up the family in its present inadequacies, would extend the possibility of social relationships that are more successfully supportive and nurturant. We should actively seek in the present to work for the kinds of social change that point towards a truly equal society, one in which women and children are truly equal with men.

NOTE

Poultanzas (1975) has also discussed class in relation to politics and in particular the nature of classes in modern, advanced capitalist societies. The relationship of women to the class structure is a complex one, which he has by no means fully explored, and I am aware that I too have merely skated over it. At times I have used the word 'class' in the sociological sense, meaning class as defined by occupation, at times in the Marxist sense to denote the relationship of the individual to the means of production. The position of the Women's Movement as regards its class structure is ambiguous. The attacks on it made by traditional economistic socialists have tended to brand it as 'middle-class' (in the sociological sense) whereas it should probably more correctly be seen as a petty-bourgeois movement, although one that is more wholly progressive than the connotations of 'petty-bourgeois' might suggest. The whole question is too important to be dealt with here, but it is certainly the case that both Marxists and sociologists in their discussions of class have tended to ignore women who once again have been defined merely by their husband's position.

References

ABBOTT, E. and BOMPASS, K. (1943) *The Woman Citizen and Social Security: A Criticism of the Proposals in the Beveridge Report as they Affect Women*. Women's Freedom League Pamphlet.

ABEL SMITH, B. and TOWNSEND, P. (1965) *The Poor and the Poorest*. London: Bell.

ADAMS, R. N. (1971) *The Nature of the Family*. In J. Goody (ed.) Harmondsworth: Penguin.

ALTHUSSER, L. (1970) *Lenin and Philosophy*. London: New Left Books.

AMERY, L. (1953) *My Political Life*, Volume II. London: Hutchinson.

ANDREWS, I. O., and HOBBS, M. A. (1918) *Economic Effects of the World War Upon Women and Children in Great Britain*. New York: Oxford University Press.

ANDRY, R. G. (1971) *Delinquency and Parental Pathology* (revised edition). London: Staples Press.

ANONYMOUS (1944) The Problem Presses. *Social Work* (Journal of the COS) 3 (1):8.

ARIÉS, P. (1973) *Centuries of Childhood*. Harmondsworth: Penguin.

ARMISTEAD, N. (ed.) (1974) *Reconstructing Social Psychology*. Harmondsworth: Penguin.

ASTBURY, B. E. (1946) The Effects of Long Separation on Family Life, and Patricia Thornton, the Lawless Child. *Social Work* 3 (2):237–41.

ATKINSON, A. B. (1969) *Poverty in Britain and the Reform of Social Security*. Cambridge: Cambridge University Press.

—— (1974) *Unequal Shares*. Harmondsworth: Penguin.

BAKER MILLER, J. (1973) *Psychoanalysis and Women*. Harmondsworth: Penguin.

BALL, S. (1896) *The Moral Aspects of Socialism*. Fabian Tract No. 72.

BANKS, J. A. and BANKS, O. (1964) *Feminism and Family Planning in Victorian England*. Liverpool: Liverpool University Press.

BARLEE, E. (1863) *A Visit to Lancashire in December 1862*. London.

BARNETT, H. (1918) *Canon Barnett, His Life, Work and Friends*. London: Murray.

BASCH, F. (1974) *Relative Creatures, Victorian Women in Society and the Novel, 1837–1876*. London: Allen Lane.

BEALES, H. L. (1952) *The Making of Social Policy*. Hobhouse Memorial Lecture, 1945. London University, London School of Economics and Political Science, Nos. 11–20. London: Oxford University Press.

BELL, N. and VOGEL, E. (eds.) (1961) *A Modern Introduction to the Family*. London: Routledge & Kegan Paul.

BENSTON, M. (1969) The Political Economy of Women's Liberation. *Monthly Review*. September.

BENYON, H. (1973) *Working for Ford*. Harmondsworth: Penguin.

BERNSTEIN, B. (1973) *Class, Codes and Control*. London: Paladin.

BEVERIDGE, W. (1909) *Unemployment A Problem of Industry*. London: Longmans.

— (1950) *Full Employment in a Free Society*. Cmnd. 7321. London: HMSO.

— (1953) *Power and Influence*. London: Hodder and Stoughton.

BLACKBURN, R. (1971) The Heath Government. *New Left Review*. No. 70, November/December.

BLACKER, C. P. (ed.) (1947) *Problem Families*. Eugenics Society.

BOOTH, W. (1890) *In Darkest England and the Way Out*. London: Salvation Army International Headquarters.

BOSANQUET, H. (1973) *Social Work in London 1869–1912*. London: Harvester Press.

BOTT, E. (1957) *Family and Social Network*. London: Tavistock Publications.

BOULDING, K. (1967) The Boundaries of Social Policy. *Social Work* 12 (1).

BOWLBY, J. A. (1963) *Child Care and the Growth of Love*. Harmondsworth: Penguin.

— (1969) *Attachment*. London: Tavistock Publications.

BRONFENBRENNER, U. (1970) *Two Worlds of Childhood, US and USSR*. New York: Russell Sage Foundation.

BROWN, G. W. (1974) Meaning Measurement and Stress of Life Events. In B. S. Dohrenwend and B. P. Dohrenwend (eds.), *Stressful Life Events: Their Nature and Effects*. New York: John Wiley.

— (1976) Depression: A Sociological Review. *Bethlem and Maudsley Gazette*. Summer.

BROWN, G. W., BHOLCHAIRI, M. N., and HARRIS, T. (1975) Social Class and Psychiatric Disturbance among Women in an Urban Population. *Sociology* 9 (2).

BROWN, G. W., HARRIS, T., and COPELAND, J. (1976) Depression and Loss. *British Journal of Psychiatry* 129.

BROWN, G. W., SKLAIR, F., HARRIS, T., and BIRLEY, J. L. T. (1973a) Life Events and Psychiatric Disorders, 1. Some Methodological Issues. *Psychological Medicine* 3 (1).

— (1973b) Life Events and Psychiatric Disorders, 2. Nature of Causal Link. *Psychological Medicine* 3 (2).

BRUCE, M. (1968) *The Coming of the Welfare State*. London: Batsford.

BULKLEY, M. E. (1914) *The Feeding of Schoolchildren*. London: Bell.

BULLOCK, A. (1967) *Life and Times of Ernest Bevin*, Volume II. London: Heinemann.

BUNBURY, H. N. (ed.) (1957) *Lloyd George's Ambulance Wagon: Being the Memoirs of William J. Braithwaite, 1911–1912.* London: Methuen.

BURN, W. L. (1964) *The Age of Equipose*. London: Unwin University Books.

CALDER, A. (1971) *The People's War*. London: Panther.

CARPENTER, M. (1853) *Juvenile Delinquents: Their Condition and Treatment*. London: W. & F. P. Cash.

CENTRAL STATISTICAL OFFICE (1974) *Social Trends*, No. 5. London: HMSO.

CHARLTON, V. and MUIR, A. (1975) Childbirth. *Spare Rib*. June.

CHOMBART DE LAUWE, M. J. (1963) *La Femme Dans La Société: Son Image dans des Différents Milieux Sociaux*. Paris: Centre National de la Recherche Scientifique.

CHRISTIAN ECONOMIC AND SOCIAL RESEARCH FOUNDATION (1957) *Young Mothers At Work*. London.

CLARKE, C. A. (1913) *The Effects of the Factory System*. London: J. M. Dent.

CLOWARD, R. and PIVEN, FOX F. (1973) *Regulating the Poor* London: Tavistock Publications.

COATES, K. and SILBURN, R. (1968) *Poverty, The Forgotten Englishman*. Hardmondsworth: Penguin.

COHEN, S. (1972) *Folk Devils and Moral Panics: The Creation of the Mods and Rockers*. London: Paladin.

COLE, G. D. H. and POSTGATE, R. (1961) *The Common People 1746–1946*. London: Methuen.

COMER, L. (1974) *Wedlocked Women*. Leeds: Feminist Books.

COMFORT, A. (1970) A Chairman's Closing Remarks. In K. Elliott (ed.), *The Family and Its Future*. Ciba Foundation Symposium. London: Churchill.

COUNTER INFORMATION SERVICE (1975) *Cutting the Welfare State*. Nottingham: CIS/CDP.

CROSLAND, A. (1958) *The Future of Socialism*. London: Jonathan Cape.

DANGERFIELD, G. (1971) *The Strange Death of Liberal England*. London: Panther.

DEACON, A. and HILL, M. (1972) The Problem of 'Surplus Women' in the Nineteenth Century: Secular and Religious Alternatives. *A Sociological Yearbook of Religion in Britain*, Volume V. London: SCM Press.

DELPHY, C. (1976) Continuities and Discontinuities in Marriage and Divorce In D. L. Barker and S. Allen *Sexual Divisions and Society: Process and Change*. London: Tavistock.

DEVINE, P. (1974) Inflation and Marxist Theory. *Marxism Today* 18 (3).

DICEY, A. V. (1905) *Lectures on the Relation Between Law and Opinion in the Nineteenth Century*. London: Macmillan.

ELLIS, K. and PETCHESKY, R. (1972) Children of the Corporate Dream: An Analysis of Day Care as a Political Issue under Capitalism. *Socialist Revolution* No. 12. January.

ENGELS, F. (1970) The Origins of the Family, Private Property and the State. In Karl Marx and Frederick Engels, *Selected Works*. London: Lawrence and Wishart.

—— (1973) *The Condition of the Working-Class in England*. Moscow: Progress Publishers.

FERGUSON, S. and FITZGERALD, H. (1949) *Social Service, UK History of the Second World War*. London: HMSO.

FERRI, E. (1976) *Growing Up in a One Parent Family*. London: NFER Publishing Company.

FINE, BEN and HARRIS, LAURENCE (1976a) The State Expenditure Debate. *New Left Review* (98), July/August.

—— (1976b) Controversial Issues in Marxist Economic Theory. In Ralph Miliband and John Saville (eds.) *The Socialist Register 1976*. London: The Merlin Press.

FINER, S. E. (1952) *The Life of Sir Edwin Chadwick*. London: Methuen.

FIRESTONE, SHULAMITH (1971) *The Dialectics of Sex*. London: Jonathan Cape.

FLETCHER, R. (1963) *The Family and Marriage in Britain*. Harmondsworth: Penguin.

FOGARTY, M., RAPOPORT, R., and RAPOPORT, T. (1971) *Sex, Career and Family*. London: PEP.

FOOT, M. (1962) *Aneurin Bevan 1897–1945*, Volume I. London: Davis Poynter.

—— (1973) *Aneurin Bevan 1945–1960*, Volume II. London: Davis Poynter.

FREUD, A. and BURLINGHAM, D. (1974) *Infants Without Families*. London: Tavistock Publications.

FREUD, S. (1950) *Collected Papers*, Volume V. London: Hogarth Press.

—— (1974) *New Introductory Lectures* (1933). Harmondsworth: Penguin.

FRIEDAN, B. (1963) *The Feminine Mystique*. London: Gollancz.

FULFORD, R. (ed.) (1964) *Dearest Child. Letters between Queen Victoria and the Princess Royal, 1858–1861*. London: Evans Bros.

GALBRAITH, J. K. (1958) *The Affluent Society*. Hardmondsworth: Penguin.

GARDINER, J. (1975a) Women and Unemployment. *Red Rag*, No. 10 (obtainable from 22. Murray Mews, London N.W.1.).

—— (1975b) Women's Domestic Labour. *New Left Review* No. 89.

GASKELL, P. (1833) *The Manufacturing Population of England*. London: Baldwin & Cradock.

GAVRON, H. (1968) *The Captive Wife*. Harmondsworth: Penguin.

GEORGE, V. (1973) *Social Security and Society*. London: Routledge & Kegan Paul.

GEORGE, V. and WILDING, P. (1972a) Social Values, Social Class and Social Policy. *Social and Economic Administration* 6 (3).

—— (1972b) *Motherless Families*. London: Routledge & Kegan Paul.

GILBERT, B. (1966) *The Evolution of National Insurance in Britain*. London: Michael Joseph.

—— (1970) *British Social Policy 1919–1939*. London: Batsford.

GOLDTHORPE, G. (1964) *The Development of Social Policy in England, 1800–1914. Transactions of the Fifth World Congress of Sociology*, Volume IV. International Sociological Association.

GOODE, W. (1971) Force and Violence in the Family. *Journal of Marriage and the Family* 33 (4):624–35, November.

GOUGH, I. (1975) State Expenditure in Advanced Capitalism. *New Left Review*, No. 92. July/August.

HALÉVY, E. (1934) *The Rise of Democracy*. London: Ernest Benn.

HAMMOND, J. L. and B. (1930) *The Age of the Chartists*. London: Longmans Green.

—— (1969) *Lord Shaftesbury*. London: Frank Cass.

HANDLER, J. (1968) The Coercive Child Care Officer. *New Society* 12 (314).

HANMER, J. (1976) Community Action, Women's Aid and the Women's Liberation Movement. In Marge Mayo (ed.), *Women in the Community*. London: Routledge & Kegan Paul.

HANNINGTON, W. (1936) *The Problems of Distressed Areas*. London: Gollancz.

HARRISON, J. (1974) *Political Economy of Housework*. CSE Bulletin. Spring.

HENRIQUES, R. (1951) *Through The Valley*. London: Reprint Society.

H.M. GOVERNMENT (1904) *Report of the Interdepartmental Committee on Physical Deterioration*. Cmnd. 2175.

—— (1942) *Report on the Social Insurance and Allied Services (Beveridge Report)*. Cmnd. 6404. London: HMSO.

—— (1944) *White Paper on Employment Policy*. Cmnd. 6527. London: HMSO.

—— (1957) *Report on the Committee on Homosexual Offences and Prostitution (Wolfenden Report)*. Cmnd. 247. London: HMSO.

—— (1959a) *Report on the Working Party on Social Workers in the Local Authority Health and Welfare Services (Younghusband Report)*. Ministry of Health. London: HMSO.

—— (1959b) *Report of the Central Advisory Council for Education – England, (Crowther Report)*, Volume I. London: HMSO.

—— (1960) *The Report of the Committee on Children and Young Persons (Ingleby Report)*. Cmnd. 1191. London: HMSO.

—— (1963) *Half Our Future (Newsom Report)*. London: HMSO.

—— (1965) *The Child, The Family and The Young Offender* (White Paper). Cmnd. 2742. London: HMSO.

—— (1967a) *Circumstances of Families*. London: HMSO.

—— (1967b) *Children and Their Primary Schools (Plowden Report)*. London: HMSO.

—— (1968) *Report on the Personal and Allied Social Services (Seebohm Report)*. Cmnd. 3703. London: HMSO.

—— (1972) *Proposals for a Tax Credit System* (Green Paper). Cmnd. 5116. London: HMSO.

—— (1974) *Report of the Committee on One Parent Families*

(Finer Report) Volumes I and II. Cmnd. 5269. London: HMSO.

—— (1975) *Report from the Select Committee on Violence in Marriage together with Proceedings of the Committee*, Volume II. London: HMSO.

HEWITT, M. (1958) *Wives and Mothers in Victorian Industry*. London: Barrie and Rockliff.

HEYWOOD, J. (1959) *Children in Care*. London: Routledge & Kegan Paul.

HICKSON, W. (1840) *Handloom Weavers Report*. Report from the Commissioners on the State of Handloom Weavers, London.

HIGHBURY AND ISLINGTON CLAIMANTS UNION (1971) *The Unsupported Mother's Handbook*. London: Crest Press.

HILL, F. (1868) *Children of the State*. London: Macmillan.

HINTON, J. (1973) *The First Shop Stewards' Movement*. London: Allen & Unwin.

HOBSBAWM, E. J. (1968a) *Industry and Empire*. Harmondsworth: Penguin.

—— (1968b) *Labouring Men*. London: Weidenfeld & Nicolson.

HOLLIS, F. (1964) *Casework: A Psycho-Social Therapy*. London: Random House.

HOLMAN, R. (1973) Poverty, Welfare Rights and Social Work. *Social Work Today* 4 (12).

HOLTBY, W. (1934) *Women and a Changing Civilisation*. London: John Lane.

HOPKINS, H. (1963) *The New Look*. London: Secker and Warburg.

HOPKINSON, T. (1971) *Picture Post 1938–1950*. Harmondsworth: Penguin.

HUNT, A. (1968) *Survey of Women's Employment*. London: HMSO.

HUNT, D. (1970) *Parents and Children in History: The Psychology of Family Life in Early Modern France*. New York: Basic Books.

HUTCHINS, L. and HARRISON, A. (1926) *A History of Factory Legislation*. London: King.

HUTT, A. (1938) *The Postwar History of the British Working Class*. London: Gollancz.

HYGIENE COMMITTEE OF THE WOMEN'S GROUP ON PUBLIC WELFARE (1942) *Our Towns*. London.

JEPHCOTT, P., SEEAR, N. and SMITH, J. H. (1962) *Married Women Working*. London: Allen & Unwin.

JOHNSON, B. S. (ed.) (1968) *The Evacuees*. London: Gollancz.

JONES, H. (ed.) (1975) *Towards a New Social Work*. London: Routledge & Kegan Paul.

JORDAN, B. (1974) *Poor Parents*. London: Routledge & Kegan Paul.

KAMM, J. (1958) *How Different From Us: A Biography of Miss Buss and Miss Beale*. London: Bodley Head.

KELLMER PRINGLE, M. (1974) *The Needs of Children: A Personal Perspective Prepared for the DHSS*. London: Hutchinson.

KEYNES, J. M. (1940) *How to Pay for the War*. London: Macmillan.

KINKAID, J. (1973) *Poverty and Equality in Britain*. Harmondsworth: Penguin.

LAING, R. D. and ESTERSON, A. (1971) *Sanity, Madness and the Family*. Harmondsworth: Penguin.

LAND, H. (1971) Women, Work and Social Security. *Journal of Social and Economic Administration* 5 (3).

—— (1976) Women: Supporters or Supported? In D. Leonard Barker and S. Allen (eds.), *Sexual Divisions and Society: Process and Change*. London: Tavistock Publications.

LASLETT, P. (1965) *The World We Have Lost*. London: Methuen.

LENIN, V. I. (1970) *What Is To Be Done, Selected Works*, Volume I. Moscow: Progress Publishers.

LEONARD, P. (1973) Towards a Paradigm for Radical Practice. In R. Bailey and M. Brake (eds.), *Radical Social Work*. London: Edward Arnold.

LESSING, D. (1966) *A Ripple from the Storm*. London: Panther.

LISTER, R. (1973) *As Man and Wife?* Poverty Research Series No. 2. London: Child Poverty Action Group.

LOFTUS, M. (1974) *Learning, Sexism and Femininity*. Red Rag No. 7.

LONGMATE, N. (1973) *How We Lived Then*. London: Arrow Books.

LOVETT, W. (1956) *Women's Mission*. Pamphlet.

LOWNDES, G. (1960) *Mary McMillan 'The Children's Champion'*. London: Museum Press.

MACBROOM, E. (1970) Socialization and Social Casework. In R. Roberts and R. H. Nee (eds.), *Theories of Social Casework.* Chicago: Chicago University Press.

MACARTHY, M. (1960) *On The Contrary.* London: Heinemann.

MACCLELLAN, D. (ed.) (1968) *Marx Before Marxism.* Harmondsworth: Penguin.

MCGREGOR, O. R. (1957) *Divorce in England, A Centenary Study.* London: Heinemann.

MCMILLAN, M. (1919) *The Nursery School.* London: Dent.

MABERLEY, A. (1948) Family Relationships. *Social Work* 5 (2).

MANTON, J. (1965) *Elizabeth Garrett Anderson.* London: Methuen.

MARRIS, P. (1958) *Widows and Their Families.* London: Routledge & Kegan Paul.

MARRIS, P. and REIN, M. (1970) *Dilemmas of Social Reform.* London: Routledge & Kegan Paul.

MARSHALL, T. H. (1965) *Social Policy.* London: Hutchinson.

MARWICK, A. (1968) *Britain in the Century of Total War.* London: Bodley Head.

—— (1973) *The Deluge.* London: Macmillan.

MARX, K. and ENGELS, F. (1970) *Selected Works.* London: Lawrence & Wishart.

MEARNS, A. (1883) *The Bitter Cry of Outcast London. An Enquiry into the Condition of the Abject Poor.* (Sometimes attributed to William Preston.) London: Congregational Union.

MILIBAND, R. (1969) *The State in Capitalist Society.* London: Weidenfeld & Nicolson.

—— (1973) *Parliamentary Socialism. A Study in the Politics of Labour.* London: Merlin Press.

MILL, J. S. (1869) *The Subjection of Women.* London: Longmans Green, Reader, and Dyer.

MILTON, N. (1973) *John Maclean.* London: Pluto Press.

MILWARD, A. S. (1970) *The Economic Effects of the Two World Wars on Britain.* London: Macmillan.

MISHRA, R. (1975) Marx and Welfare. *The Sociological Review* 23 (2):287–313.

MITCHELL, J. (1971) *Women's Estate.* Harmondsworth: Penguin.

MOBERLEY BELL, E. (1942) *Octavia Hill*. London: Constable.

MORTON, P. (1970) Women's Work is Never Done. *Leviathan*.

MYRDAL, A. and KLEIN, V. (1956) *Women's Two Roles*. London: Routledge & Kegan Paul.

NSPCC (1974) Yo Yo Children: A Study of Twenty-Three Violent Matrimonial Cases. London: NSPCC.

NUTTALL, J. (1970) *Bomb Culture*. London: Paladin.

OAKLEY, A. (1975) The Trap of Medicalised Motherhood. *New Society* 34 (689)

PADLEY, R. and COLE, M. (eds.) (1940) *Evacuation Survey: A Report to the Fabian Society*. London: George Routledge.

PANKHURST, S. (1911) *The Suffragette*. London: Gay & Hancock.

—— (1930) *Save the Mothers*. London: A. A. Knopf.

—— (1931) *The Suffragette Movement*. London: Longmans.

PASHLEY, R. (1855) *Pauperism and Poor Laws*. London.

PAUL, W. (1917) *The State: Its Origin and Function*. Glasgow: Socialist Labour Press.

PEARSON, G. (1973) Social Work as the Privatised Solution of Public Ills. *British Journal of Social Work* 3 (2).

PERKIN, H. (1969) *The Origins of Modern English Society, 1780–1880*. London: Methuen.

PINCHBECK, I. (1930) *Women Workers and the Industrial Revolution, 1750–1850*. Oxford: Oxford University Press.

PINCHBECK, I. and HEWITT, M. (1973) *Children in English Society*, Volume II. London: Routledge & Kegan Paul.

PINCUS, A. and MINAHAN, A. (1973) *Social Work Practice: Model and Method*. Ithaca, Ill.: F. E. Peacock Publishers.

PINCUS, L. (ed.) (1953) *Social Casework in Marital Problems*. London: Tavistock Publications.

PINKER, R. (1971) *Social Theory and Social Policy*. London: Heinemann.

POLITICAL AND ECONOMIC PLANNING (1952) *Government and Industry*. London: PEP.

POLLARD, S. (1969) *The Development of the British Economy, 1914–1967*. London: Edward Arnold.

POULANTZAS, N. (1972) The Problem of the Capitalist State. In R. Blackburn (ed.), *Ideology in Social Science*. London: Fontana/Collins.

—— (1973) *Political Power and Social Classes*. London: New Left Books.

—— (1975) *Classes in Contemporary Capitalism*. London: New Left Books.

POWELL, E. and MACLEOD, I. (1952) *The Social Services, Needs and Means*. London: Conservative Central Office.

POWER COBBE, F. (1869) The Final Cause of Women. In Josephine Butler (ed.), *Woman's Work and Woman's Culture*. London: Macmillan.

—— (1878) Wife Torture in England. *Contemporary Review* xxxii: 55–87.

—— (1881) *The Duties of Women: A Course of Lectures*. London and Edinburgh: Williams and Norgate.

RAMELSON, M. (1965) *The Petticoat Rebellion*. London: Lawrence and Wishart.

RAPOPORT, R. and RAPOPORT, R. (1971) *Dual Career Families*. Harmondsworth: Penguin.

RATHBONE, E. (1913) *Report on the Conditions of Widows under the Poor Law In Liverpool*. Presented to the Annual Meeting of the Liverpool Women's Industrial Council, December.

RICHTER, M. (1964) *The Politics of Conscience: T. H. Green and His Age*. London: Weidenfeld & Nicolson.

ROBERTS, D. (1960) *Victorian Origins of the British Welfare State*. Yale: Yale University Press.

ROGOW, A. A. (1955) *The Labour Government and British Industry, 1945–1951*. Oxford: Oxford University Press.

ROSE, H. (1972) *Up Against the Welfare State*. Socialist Register.

ROSE, M. E. (1972) *The Relief of Poverty, 1834–1914*. London: Macmillan.

ROSEN, A. (1974) *Rise Up Women!: The Militant Campaign of the Women's Social and Political Union, 1903–1914*. London: Routledge & Kegan Paul.

ROSSER, C. and HARRIS, T. (1965) *The Family and Social Change: A Study of Family and Kinship in a South Wales Town*. London: Routledge & Kegan Paul.

ROWBOTHAM, S. (1973) *Women's Consciousness, Man's World*. Harmondsworth: Penguin.

ROWNTREE, S. (1901) *Poverty: A Study of Town Life*. London: Macmillan.

—— (1936) *The Human Needs of Labour*. London.

—— (1941) *Poverty and Progress: A Second Social Survey of York*. London: Longmans.

—— (1951) *Poverty and the Welfare State: A Third Social Survey of York dealing with Economic Questions*. London: Longmans.

RUSKIN, J. (1865) *Sesame and Lilies*. London.

RUTTER, M. (ed.) (1972) *Maternal Deprivation Reassessed*. Harmondsworth: Penguin.

SAVILLE, J. (1958) The Welfare State, An Historical Approach. *The New Reasoner*, No. 3.

SECOMBE, W. (1974) *The Housewife and Her Labour under Capitalism*. *New Left Review*, No. 83.

SEED, P. (1973) *The Expansion of Social Work*. London: Routledge & Kegan Paul.

SHONFIELD, A. (1958) *British Economic Policy Since the War*. Harmondsworth: Penguin.

—— (1976) *Cycles of Disadvantage*. London: Heinemann.

SIMON, B. (1965) *Education and the Labour Movement*. London: Lawrence and Wishart.

SISSONS, M. and FRENCH, P. (1963) *The Age of Austerity*. Harmondsworth: Penguin.

SLATER, E. and WOODSIDE, M. (1951) *Patterns of Marriage*. London: Cassel.

SMELSER, N. (1969) *Social Change in the Industrial Revolution*. London: Routledge & Kegan Paul.

SOCIALIST MEDICAL ASSOCIATION (1964) *A Socialist View of Social Work*. Pamphlet.

SPRING RICE, M. (1939) *Working Class Wives*. Harmondsworth: Penguin.

STEDMAN JONES, G. (1971) *Outcast London*. Oxford: Oxford University Press.

STEVENSON, O. (1972) *Claimant or Client*. London: Allen & Unwin.

STEWART, M. (1971) *Keynes and After*. Harmondsworth: Penguin.

STOCKS, M. (1949) *Eleanor Rathbone*. London: Gollancz.

—— (1970) *My Commonplace Book*. London: Peter Davies.

STRACHEY, R. (1928) *The Cause*. London: Bell.

STREATHER, J. and WEIR, S. (1974) *Social Insecurity: Single*

Mothers on Benefit. Poverty Pamphlet No. 16. London: Child Poverty Action Group.

THOMPSON, E. P. (1968) *The Making of the English Working Class*. Harmondsworth: Penguin.

THOMPSON, D. (1958) Reply to John Saville. *The New Reasoner*, No. 4.

THOMPSON, F. (1973) *Lark Rise to Candleford*. Harmondsworth: Penguin.

TITMUSS, R. M. (1950) *Problems of Social Policy, UK (Cabinet Office) History of the Second World War*. UK Civil Service Series. London: HMSO.

—— (1962) *Income Distribution and Social Change*. London: Allen & Unwin.

—— (1963) *Essays on the Welfare State*. London: Allen & Unwin.

—— (1968) *Commitment to Welfare*. London: Allen & Unwin.

TOWNSEND, P. (1957) *The Family Life of Old People*. London: Routledge & Kegan Paul.

—— (1958) A Society for People. In N. Mackenzie (ed.), *Conviction*. St. Albans: McGibbon & Kee.

TWINING, L. (1880) *Workhouse Visiting and Management*. London: Routledge & Kegan Paul.

—— (1893) *Recollections of Life and Work*. London: Edward Arnold.

VAIZEY, J. (1962) *Education For Tomorrow*. Harmondsworth: Penguin.

WARREN, B. (1972) Capitalist Planning and the State. *New Left Review*, No. 72.

WEBB, B. (1926) Our Partnership. London: Longmans.

WEBB, S. (1907) The Decline of the Birthrate. *Fabian Tract*, No. 131.

—— (1969) *My Apprenticeship*. Harmondsworth: Penguin.

WEINBERGER, P. E. (ed.) (1975) *Perspectives on Social Welfare*. New York: Macmillan.

WEIR, A. (1975) In Sandra Allen, Lee Sanders, and Jan Wallis (eds.) *Conditions of Illusion*. Leeds: Feminist Books.

—— (1976) Battered Women. In Marge Mayo (ed.), *Women in the Community*. London: Routledge & Kegan Paul.

WESTERGAARD, J. and RESLER, H. (1975) *Class in a Capitalist Society*. London: Heinemann.

WHITE, A. (1901) *Efficiency and Empire*. London: Methuen.

WILDEBLOOD, P. (1958) *Against the Law*. Harmondsworth: Penguin.

WILSON, E. (1975) Margaret Thatcher. *Red Rag*, No. 9.

WISE, A. (1972) *Women and the Struggle for Workers' Control*. Nottingham: Spokesman Pamphlet.

WOODROOFE, K. (1962) *From Charity to Social Work*. London: Routledge & Kegan Paul.

WOOTTON, B. (1959) *Social Science and Social Pathology*. London: Routledge & Kegan Paul.

WYNN, M. (1971) *Family Policy*. Harmondsworth: Penguin.

YOUNG, M. (ed.) (1974) *Poverty Report*. London: Maurice Temple Smith.

—— (ed.) (1975) *Poverty Report*. London: Maurice Temple Smith.

YOUNG, M. and WILLMOTT, P. (1958) *Family and Kinship in East London*. London: Routledge & Kegan Paul.

YOUNGHUSBAND, E. (ed.) (1965) *Social Work with Families*. London: Allen & Unwin.

YUDKIN, S. and HOLME, A. (1963) *Working Mothers and Their Children*. London: Michael Joseph.

ZELDIN, T. (1973) *France 1848–1945*, Volume I. Oxford: Oxford University Press.

Subject Index

abortion, 169, 170, 179, 181–2
'affluent society', 75–6

battered women, 26, 173
  and the police, 174
  and social workers, 173–4
Beveridge Report, 140, 141, 142,
  143, 148–54
birth control, 117
  repressive fertility control, 69–
  70
birth rate, 74, 158
  compression of fertility, 171–2
  declining birth rate, 101–2, 133,
  155, 179

'Captive Wife, The', 160–2

'Case Con', 92
casework, 28, 36–7, 50–1, 84, 86,
  87
centralism,
  growth of, 29
charity, 49
Charity Organisation Society, 49–
  51, 86, 104
Chartists,
  attitude to women, 25–6
childbirth, 123, 181
childcare, 95, 96, 123, 134, 139,
  154, 155, 158, 182, 183
  in the nineteenth century,
  45–6
  see also Mia Kellmer Pringle,
  John Bowlby

childhood,
    changing ideas of, 15–17, 19–20
Children & Young Persons Act,
    1969, 88–9, 175
Christian Socialists, 32, 47
class struggle, 31
    and the bourgeois state, 11
    and the white-collar sector,
    179–81
cohabitation ruling, 13, 80–1, 153
collectivism vs. socialism, 30–1
Contagious Diseases Acts (1864–
    69),
    campaign against, 56–7

'dilution of labour', 129–30, 131
'diswelfares', 74–5, 98

economism, 10–11, 37, 38, 182
equal pay, 121, 131–2, 162, 165,
    170
Equal Pay Act (1970), 8, 162, 170
evacuation, 136–9

Fabians, fabianism, 30–2, 102
Factory Acts, factory legislation,
    28, 38, 98
family, 8–9, 84, 179
    decline in family size, 133, 171–
    2
    'dual career' families, 166–8
    and the poor law, 54–5
    'problem families', 37, 69, 77–8,
    138–9
    socialist feminist critique of
    186–7
    sociologists' views on, 63–4, 65,
    state intervention in, 29, 35, 40,
    67, 93, 96, 101, 107–9, 124–5,
    153, 178, 179, 183
    supportive emotional function
    of, 176
family allowances, 34, 95, 120–2,
    151
    attitude of working class to,
    140–1

Family Income Supplement, 93
feminism,
    in the inter-war period, 34, 117,
    121–2
    in the nineteenth century,
    55–6, 57–8, 59
    in the 1950s, 60, 61
    see also Women's Liberation
    Movement, Suffragettes
Finer Report, 24–5, 68, 69, 97, 153,
    172
functionalist theory of the Wel-
    fare State, 35–6
full employment economic pol-
    icy, 34–5

German social policy,
    influence of, 33, 103

homosexuality, 67, 87

incomes policy, 146–7
individualism, 28, 51
infant mortality,
    and Victorian welfare meas-
    ures, 45–7
Interdepartmental Committee on
    Physical Deterioration (1904),
    101

Keynesian economic policy,
    142–3

labour control,
    during First World War, 103,
    127–8, 129
    during Second World War,
    128–9, 131
Labour government (1945–51),
    144–7
Labour Party,
    victory, 1945, 144–5
Lesbianism, 169
Libertarianism, 38–9
Liberal reforms 1906–11, 33, 103,
    105–6

Malthusian doctrine, 16, 39
marriage, 24, 177
   anxiety about breakdown of,
     172–3
   assumptions of women's de-
     pendence in, 81, 152–4
   increased popularity of, 171
   'marriage as a career', 160
   'partnership' marriage, 64
   violence in marriage, 26, 173,
     185
   see also National Women's Aid
     Federation
maternity benefit, 151, 153
maternity leave, 46–7
Mental Health Act (1959), 89–90
midwives, 123–4
motherhood,
   financial reward for, 94, 103
     (see also family allowances)
   ideology of, 17, 22, 43, 110,
     151–2
   see also John Bowlby, S. Freud,
     Mia Kellmer Pringle

National Federation of Women
   Workers, 129, 133
'national efficiency',
   ideology of, 30, 100–3, 109, 120
National Insurance Act 1911,
   105–6
National Women's Aid Federation, 174–5
Newsom Report (1963), 82–3
nurseries,
   after the Second World War,
     97, 154
   in the nineteenth century, 46
   in wartime, 134–5, 139
   Plowden Report, 83

Old Age Pensions Act (1908), 106

'Permissive Society', the, 68, 71–2
Poor Law, 28–9, 30, 98, 108, 153
   Royal Commission on (1905–9),
     103–5

and women and children, 52–5
population control, 69, 102–3
poverty, 29, 96,
   'disappearance' cf, 75–8
   in the late nineteenth century,
     99–100
   women and, 78–80
psychoanalytic theory, 84–8,
   156–7

school meals,
   origin of legislation on, 106–9
Seebohm Report (1968), 90, 91, 92
Settlement Movement, 32, 100
Sex Discrimination Act (1975), 8,
   162, 170
sexism, 71–2, 118, 182, 183, 185
sexuality, ideas on women's
   in the inter-war period, 117–18
   in the nineteenth century,
     24–5, 43, 45, 57
   in the 1950s, 65–7
   in the 1960s, 68, 70, 161–2
'social wage', 73–4
social work,
   in the USA, 84–6, 90
   'radical social work', 37, 92
   theories underlying, 10, 28,
     36–7, 84–90
   see also casework
social workers,
   attitudes towards battered
     wives and children, 173–4
   and management of working-
     class families, 47, 83–4, 88–9,
     156–8, 166 see also family,
     state intervention in
   professionalization of, 111
   repolitization of, 92
   repressive role of, 13, 83–4, 91
   and the Second World War,
     139–40
'student unrest', 10, 159
Suffragettes, 111, 112, 115

unemployment, 103, 119

and prostitution, 57
and women 162–3
unemployment insurance, 119
and women 119–20, 150
universalism, 77
attacks on 77–8

welfare work, 133
welfarism, 28, 29–30, 128, 178
womanhood, ideal of, 22–4, 25–6,
  43, 44, 83, 112
women,
  and the Beveridge Report, 149–
  54
  bourgeois women, 22, 25, 56
  and education, 81–3, 159–60,
  162
  and industrialization, 18–26
  and the NHS, 180–1
  and the reproduction of the
  workforce, 8
  and unpaid domestic labour,
  176–8

women workers,
  after the Second World War,
  155–6, 163–4, 170
  and the First World War, 117,
  129–35
  and the Second World War,
  131–3, 134
  in the nineteenth century, 18–
  21, 47
  in the professions, 156, 160,
  164–5
  in the public sector, 180–1
  and unemployment, 162–3
  working mothers, 62–3, 76, 83,
  151, 163, 179
Women's Liberation Movement,
  10, 11, 14, 39, 59, 92, 162, 171,
  175, 182–6, 179
  Six demands of, 41
Working Women's Charter, 170

Younghusband Report, 89

Joseph, Sir Keith, 93
Jordan, Bill, 96

Keynes, John Maynard, 142

Laing, R. D., 71
Lessing, Doris, 175
Loch, C. S., 50, 51

MacDonald, James Ramsay and
  Margaret, 115

Nixon, Richard, 167

Pankhurst, Christabel, 25
Pankhurst, Sylvia, 34, 123, 135,
  175
Pizzey, Erin, 174
Pringle, Mia Kellmer, 93–5, 96,
  172

Poulantzas, Nicos, 10, 11, 13, 178

Rathbone, Eleanor, 34, 120–2
Rowntree, B. Seebohm, 75, 76,
  114–15, 149
Ruskin, John, 22, 48, 49

Saville, John, 178

Thompson, Dorothy, 178
Titmuss, Richard, 105, 114, 126,
  139, 140, 160, 170
Townsend, Peter, 11
Twining, Louisa, 52–4, 110

Webb, Beatrice, 30, 40–1, 112, 113
Webb, Sidney, 30, 103
  see also Fabians
Wynn, Margaret, 95–6

Author Index

Althusser, Louis, 13, 15

Beveridge, William, 8, 32, 75,
102, 103, 119, 121, 127, 128,
129, 147, 155,
see also Beveridge Report
Bevin, Ernest, 128-9, 131, 132
Bosanquet, Helen, 51, 104
Boulding, Kenneth, 12
Bowlby, John, 64-5, 79, 94, 96-7,
137-8, 165
Boyd Orr, John, 120, 122
Butler, Josephine, 56-7, 161

Carpenter, Mary, 54-5, 58
Chamberlain, Joseph, 30

Dicey, A. V., 28, 35

Engels, Frederick, 19, 44, 182-5

Firestone, Shulamith, 184
Freud, Sigmund, 65, 85, 156, 157,
161

Gardiner, Jean, 162, 163, 164
Garrett Anderson, Elizabeth, 47,
57
Gavron, Hannah, 160-2
Goldberg, E. M., 166
Green, T. H., 32

Hannington, Wal, 122
Hill, Florence, 55
Hill, Octavia, 48-9, 51, 111, 113
Holtby, Winifred, 118